I0569218

SELF -PRESERVATION

choosing to thrive

TIM ANDERSON

Self Preservation: Choosing to Thrive by Tim Anderson
Copyright © 2026 by Original Strength Systems, LLC.

All rights reserved.

Cover design and interior by Stewart A. Williams

Published by OS Press, Fuquay-Varina, NC

Paperback
ISBN: 978-1-963675-17-7

eBook
ISBN: 978-1-963675-18-4

Library of Congress Number available upon request.

All rights reserved. Except in the case of brief quotations embodied in critical articles and reviews, no portion of this book may be reproduced, stored in a retrieval system, or transmitted in any form or by any means; electronic, mechanical, photocopy, recording, scanning, or other, without the prior written permission from the author. For permission to copy, send requests to Original Strength Systems, LLC, 212 S Main Street, Fuquay-Varina, NC 27526.

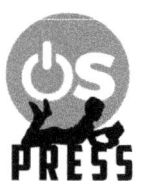

CONTENTS

INTRODUCTION

If you've ever been on a plane, you're probably familiar with the safety presentation involving the oxygen masks. Different airlines word it differently, but the gist is universal, and it goes something like this:

"In the unlikely event of an emergency...If cabin oxygen levels drop below the required level, oxygen masks will drop from the overhead lockers. Place the mask over your face and secure it by pulling the straps tightly. Do not worry if the bag does not inflate; you are still getting oxygen. Put your mask on before attempting to help someone else with theirs."

Have you ever pondered, or perhaps experienced this scenario, and thought about what it would be like to have to put on your own oxygen mask or try to help someone else put on theirs? Or, thought that you could probably manage to help someone else put their mask on first, and then put your mask on in time to save yourself?

There is no doubt that in a casual, non-stressful situation, you could easily help another person put on their mask, then put on yours. With practice, if you were to practice such a thing, you could likely help someone else put on their mask and don your mask in less than 5 seconds. And while practice is beneficial, sometimes the gravity of an emergency can overwhelm us. After all, it can be hard to navigate through the adrenaline dump of a life-or-death situation. In a genuine emergency, it can be hard to control your thoughts. Often, emergencies can make it hard to control your own body. Emergencies change the game and influence whether we react or respond. They put the unimaginable weights of stress on your shoulders, on your lungs, and on your mental and emotional faculties.

This is why airlines suggest securing your mask first. If you can do that, you'll likely be able to help many of the passengers around you. But did you notice the most essential instruction in the safety brief? "Do not worry..." Mask or no mask, the bag fills, or it doesn't, but just don't worry. Worry hijacks your mind and alters your mental and physical destination for the worse. Worry sabotages you.

Anyway, "put your mask on first..." If you fumble around too long in a highly stressed state, you're going to run out of time and air. You're likely going to succumb to the extreme form of worry and panic. At that point, you will no longer be helpful to anyone, and you may even become a detriment to everyone.

There is something to be said for self-preservation, or having the ability to preserve your life. If you can take care of yourself, you'll be able to take care of those around you. If you can't take care of yourself, you're going to drain those around you, and you may even take them down with you.

We see daily examples of this everywhere we look. People who age far too quickly and end up in rest homes often need the concerted care of a team. People who become too weak to get out of bed or off the floor often need help from family members or emergency responders. In a broader sense, a society where the majority of the population is overweight or suffering from some type of "itis" strains the entire society through increased costs of health care, insurance, and pharmaceuticals. When someone can't preserve their life, they will drain, strain, and weigh others down with them. It happens.

The purpose of this book is to help you achieve a rich, full life through learning True Self preservation skills. Not only that, but if you can learn to preserve your true life, you'll have the strength, energy, and **desire** to help someone else in need of finding theirs. It's true. When you feel good, you can't help but want to help others feel good, too.

That's the point. You're designed to live a robust, "feel-good" life; to be a guide and a help to those around you. But if you're not able to do that, your life is going to shrink and close in on you; it will slip away from you. If that happens, your life is going to start clawing at the lives of those around you.

You may or may not know this, but a drowning person often drowns the "Good Samaritans" who try to help them. They don't mean to, but they panic, and they thrash and fight their would-be rescuers. They cannot navigate through their emergency; they don't have the skills (they don't know how to swim). Fear sets in, and they take others with them.

Here's the thing, life IS an emergency. It is emergent; in the process of coming into being. Every moment is brand new. Life is like a wave. If we can navigate it and surf it, we can live an extraordinary life that brings us joy; it can also be a life that brings joy to those around us. But if we can't surf it, if we get pulled under by it or even miss it, we'll eventually drown and drag others down with us.

None of us really wants that.

We want to ride the wave of life and ride it well. To do this, we need to learn how to swim and surf; we need to learn how to preserve our lives.

In the following pages, we will examine the keys to true self-preservation. You should know, this is not a selfish endeavor. It's quite the opposite, even upside down from it. In my mind, self-preservation is the key to finding and enjoying life. It's about restoring and preserving the self you were created to be; it leads to the life you were meant to live —a life free of worry and full of joy.

If you've ever felt weighed down, maybe like you were sinking or drowning, or like you just couldn't breathe, you can change all of that. You can preserve or restore your true self, your life. You can feel good again, or even for the first time. You can also be a help to those around you who may be experiencing the same struggles. When you start doing that, you'll discover a "feel-good" state of being like you've never known. It feels ah-mazing to be able to help others. There's nothing more fulfilling and invigorating.

Anyway, hopefully all of this will make sense by the end of the book. For now, if you're willing and able, let's put on our oxygen masks, turn the page, and breathe.

Special Note:

Movement and Exercise have risks associated with them. Research shows they can lead to being stronger, healthier, and happier. However, they can also lead to injuries or even death. It happens.

You should also know that doing nothing also has risks associated with it. Research shows that being sedentary can lead to sickness, weakness, frailty, depression, and anxiety. It can also make you more injury-prone and hasten your destination towards death. It happens.

Before beginning any exercise program, consult your trusted family physician. You should also consult your trusted family physician before engaging in any sedentary lifestyle.

THE ONE THING

In the human body, in the known universe for that matter, everything affects everything. That means your body is so interconnected and intricately designed that anything that happens to it, or in it, affects the whole of it. Nothing about you works in isolation. Everything affects everything, and therefore everything matters. It makes sense then that if everything affects everything, then one thing affects everything. And there is one thing you do that affects the whole of you. This one thing is perhaps the most important and systemically influential thing you do: Breathing.

Breathing is so important that I've written about it in 13 different books. With each of those attempts, I have been able to better explain the importance and benefits of proper breathing. With this book, I hope to nail it. Practice strengthens us and makes us better, right?

This book is about self-preservation: saving ourselves so we can help "save" (serve) others. In the area of self-preservation, breathing is of the utmost importance. It is the one thing that matters most because it is the foundation of every other aspect of our being.

Look at this Hierarchy of Physiology diagram. Breathing upholds everything.

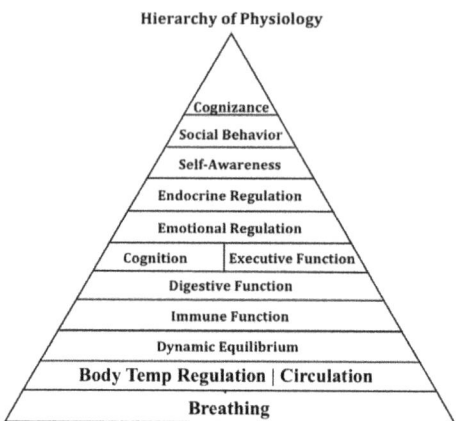

Hierarchy of Physiology

Cognizance
Social Behavior
Self-Awareness
Endocrine Regulation
Emotional Regulation
Cognition | Executive Function
Digestive Function
Immune Function
Dynamic Equilibrium
Body Temp Regulation | Circulation
Breathing

How you breathe even affects how your genes express themselves. If you could master one thing and perfect one movement to optimize your physical health, emotional state, and life's experiences, it should be breathing.

In Original Strength courses, we teach that there are three pillars of human movement:

1) Breathing the way you were designed to breathe.
2) Activating your vestibular system.
3) Engaging in your gait pattern.

But I'm willing to take this much further. There is one foundation to *being,* and that is breathing. Breath truly is life. Not just because it's how we take in oxygen, but because the act of it is how we engage in and respond to life.

If we want to preserve, enjoy, and maximize our lives, it is paramount that we breathe the way we were designed to. But it's equally paramount that we explore our breath and learn to harness its powers. There are times in life when, if we are mindful and intentional, we can use our breath to elevate ourselves out of stressful situations, or even perilous ones. There are also times in life where we can harness our breath to navigate emotionally charged conversations or even mitigate our fears. And there are times in life where we can use our breath to heal our bodies and our souls.

I know you know this, but breathing is not just breathing. It is absolute life to us. It's the one thing that leads to everything, "good" or "bad." This is why I say if you could just master one movement, master this one. Breathe within your design to optimize your physical, mental, and emotional health, but also learn to design your life with your breath.

Let's walk through this together.

The Design of Breath

Breath is the foundation of being, and we are designed to breathe a certain way. I've written extensively about this in other books, so I'll just give you a recap here. The human baby is born as an obligate nasal breather. This means that the human infant is physiologically designed to breathe exclusively through its nose. This remains the case for the first several months of life, until compensations are learned through experiences such as sickness, injury, or fear.

> Nasal breathing is our design. It leads to optimal function of the human body.

Nasal breathing is our design. It leads to optimal function of the human body. It is the Breath of Peace. Mouth breathing is a compensatory breathing pattern. It changes (affects) everything about our body in a negative way. It is the Breath of Fear.

As once obligate nasal breathers, we kept our tongues rested on the roof of our mouths, pulled air all the way down into our lungs with our diaphragm, and maintained our autonomic nervous system in its default parasympathetic state. We were at peace physically, mentally, and emotionally. If you look at a newborn baby's face, you know this is true.

As compensatory mouth breathers, we lose control of our tongues, we typically corral air to the upper part of our lungs with our smaller accessory breathing muscles, and we keep our autonomic nervous system in its emergency sympathetic state. This is a state of physical stress, mental limitation, and emotional fear and anxiety. If you look at the average adult mouth breather's face, you know this is also true.

Physiologically, your breath is the key to overall well-being. Remember, everything affects everything. How you move (how you breathe) affects how you think and how you feel. Your thoughts and feelings influence how you breathe. If you are moving (breathing) optimally, you have more access to thinking and feeling optimally as well. If you breathe well, you are more likely to experience peace, love, joy, creativity, and rational thinking. Your default state, your affect, will be pleasant; you'll enjoy being in your own skin. In other words, you'll enjoy being you. This is a layer of self-preservation. You're preserving the state of You that you were intended to be. The You that can live the life you want to live.

I have to tell you, the design of breath is simply beyond brilliant. And once you see it, you can't unsee it. In an attempt to share my awe with you, let me tell you just a little bit about how you were born to breathe. (I'm not sure anyone is capable of fully revealing all the wonder of breath.)

The Narrow Way

"Enter through the narrow gate; for the gate is wide and the way is broad that leads to destruction, and there are many who enter through it. For the gate is narrow and the way is constricted that leads to life, and there are few who find it."

–MATTHEW 7:13-14 NKJV

As I mentioned above, we are born nasal breathers. As it turns out, your nasal passages are narrower than your oral passages. It requires more effort, creates more turbulence, and generates more intra-abdominal pressure when we breathe in and out of our noses. In other words, nasal breathing literally makes you stronger. It creates strength and is the ultimate core strengthener.

Nasal breathing strengthens us from the inside out

That's right, nasal breathing strengthens your "core" breathing muscles, also known as your "inner-core" muscles. Your inner core muscles include the diaphragm, transverse abdominal muscles, pelvic floor, and multifidi. These muscles are responsible for stabilizing your spine and providing a foundation of strength to support your movements. They are like the rock that the wise man built his house upon. When we are breathing within our design, these muscles dance together and function properly. They allow us to move fluidly, maintain optimal posture, and perform with strength and power. They also help to protect us from injury.

Nasal breathing strengthens us from the inside out. It is interconnected with our diaphragms, serving as our postural support and intra-thoracic pressure valves. Through breathing in and out of our small nasal passages and exercising our diaphragms, we become rooted, or solid, in our bodies. I know this may be confusing, but our pelvic floor, diaphragm, vocal cords, and tongue act as lids; they help us contain pressure, which keeps us resilient and capable of generating huge amounts of power.

When our tongue is in place on the roof of our mouth, and we breathe through our nose, our diaphragm and pelvic floor muscles descend and ascend together, and our transverse abdominal muscles expand and contract with them. These muscles create a type of pressurized cylinder in our center. Additionally, our tongue and vocal cords help prevent this internal pressure from leaking out. Try this for yourself. Compare breathing through your nose and breathing through your mouth. You can feel the difference in pressure in your center when breathing through your nose versus your mouth. Do you also notice the difference in your posture? Nasal breathing puts "juice" in your posture; it strengthens your structure. Mouth breathing allows the "juice" to escape, weakening your structure.

The Air We Breathe

"The air goes where it wishes, and you hear the sound of it, you can even feel it, but you cannot tell where it comes from and where it goes."

–THE CARPENTER

Obviously, breathing is the process by which we take in oxygen (O2) and release carbon dioxide (CO2). Have you ever pondered this, I mean, the broader design of breath? Think of the wonder for just one second. We need oxygen to survive. Plants produce oxygen. Plants need carbon dioxide to survive. We, along with other animals, produce carbon dioxide. The balance of this, the interdependence of the existence of all living things, is staggering. One was made for the other, and the other was made for one. There is a design and a purpose for all created things. It's just awe-inspiring.

Anyway, the air we breathe contains just the right amount of oxygen, 21%. If you've read my book, *Discovering You*, you know that there's something special about the number 21; it's the perfect number. If the air we breathe were to have less than 21% oxygen, we would become hypoxic, get sick, and even die. If the air we breathe were to have more than 21% we could get oxygen toxicity, get sick, and even die. 21%, no more, no less.

Somehow, this perfect percentage of oxygen is extracted from the air by the alveoli in our lungs when we inhale. Oxygen is then picked up by our red blood cells and carried to all our tissues. It keeps every cell in our bodies alive. If our lungs were to become compromised and unable to extract enough oxygen from the air, it could lead to hypoxia, respiratory failure, and ultimately death - just like breathing in air that had less than 21% oxygen in it.

What if I told you that mouth breathing was like a form of self-induced lung compromise? When people breathe in through their mouths, they tend to only breathe into the upper portion of their lungs. This happens because they are not fully utilizing their diaphragm to draw air down into the lower parts of their lungs. Instead, they are relying on their accessory breathing muscles, also known as their emergency breathing muscles. Air is not water; it's air. What I mean by that is that air fills the spaces it is pulled into, but it is not affected by gravity the same way a liquid is. When poured into a container, a liquid will fill the container from the bottom to the top. If you pour air into a container, where does it go? Nowhere, because you can't really pour air into a container. You have to pull it in, you have to invite it in. Our inhalation is an invitation for air to enter our lungs. But if we only invite air to the top of our lungs, that is where it will go.

You might be thinking, "Yeah, so we are only using the alveoli in the top portion of our lungs. Is that such a big deal?" The answer to that is ABSOLUTELY, especially when you consider that two-thirds of the alveoli in our lungs are located at the bottom of our lungs. Mouth breathers are only flirting with one-third of their oxygen-exchanging capacity. This forces them to work harder to deliver oxygen to all their tissues; they must breathe faster, and their hearts must pump faster. Do you know what this reinforces for the brain? **"I am in danger," "Something is wrong," "I am not safe."**

Air is life to us, but so is how we invite it in. We are designed to fill all of our lungs with air, especially the bottom of our lungs. When we breathe in through our nose, it increases the likelihood that this will happen naturally. Remember, the nasal passages are narrower than the mouth passage. It requires more effort, more pull; a larger "invitation" is needed when we breathe in through our nose. This greater effort requires more work from the diaphragm and invites air deeper into our lungs, where our alveoli can extract more oxygen to supply our body's tissues.

When we take in adequate air by filling our lungs, we naturally breathe slower, and our heart doesn't have to work as hard because we are getting adequate oxygen to our tissues. Our brain is always monitoring these things. When we receive adequate oxygen and breathe through our nose, our brain signals that we are safe and all is well. This allows the body to thrive in a state of ease and balance.

There's another thing that a good inhale provides for us; it allows us to have a good exhale. When we breathe shallowly, we also exhale shallowly. When we don't fully exhale, we retain carbon dioxide in our lungs. This, again, makes it more challenging to take in the oxygen we need, and we end up breathing faster and more shallowly. Our brain freaks out, and then we get anxious or even panic (in extreme cases).

Not only do we want to invite air into the depths of our lungs, but we also want to usher it out. We achieve this through adequate exhalation, when our diaphragm and rib cage return to their natural resting position. If we exhale through our nasal passages, the pressure is higher than if we exhale through our mouth passages. The higher pressure from nasal exhalation also increases the time it takes to "usher" the air out of our lungs. Longer exhalations tell the brain, "**I'm very safe.**" They also help the body let go of tension, but we'll talk about that later.

The point is, if we breathe the way we were born to breathe, we are taking full advantage of our design to extract the right amount of oxygen our body needs from the exact right amount of oxygen that is in the air—the right amount for life, for our life, to be optimally lived.

Can you see the brilliance of the design yet? If not, just wait, there's more.

A Shield of Protection

Nasal Breathing also protects us, physically. When we breathe through our nose, we mix the outside air with nitric oxide, a gas we produce in our sinus cavities. Nitric oxide is a wonder gas. It is anti-viral and anti-bacterial. One of its purposes is to kill harmful pathogens in the air we breathe. When we breathe through our mouths, we bypass this gas and expose our bodies to these would-be attackers. Incidentally, nitric oxide is also a vasodilator, helping to keep our heart and blood vessels healthy. It is the reason men love viagra.

However, nitric oxide also contributes to neuroplasticity, our brains' ability to form new neural connections and repair older ones. Breathing through our noses literally keeps our brain, heart, and lungs healthy and resilient.

Incidentally, humming helps our body generate even more nitric oxide, according to some sources, up to 15 times more. Just a heads up in case you can't make it to the drug store. Use this information as you see fit!

All actual jokes aside, let's also consider the nasal passages themselves. They are filled with hair, mucus, and moisture. They condition the air we breathe, warming it and moisturizing it. They also filter particulate matter from the air. This is all part of the design to protect our lungs. The nasal passages keep pollutants out and condition the air, helping prevent the lungs from being "assaulted" by cold, dry, dirty air.

> Every breath you take sends one of two messages to your brain: "I am safe," or "I am not safe."

When we breathe through our mouths, none of this happens. We therefore force our bodies to work harder by compromising the immune system, allowing harmful substances to enter our lungs.

The Breath of Peace

Perhaps the biggest and best reason to breathe within your design is due to the state of being your breath determines. As I mentioned earlier, breathing through our nose is like the breath of peace and tranquility. It keeps us in our parasympathetic, rest-and-be state. Breathing through our mouths is like the breath of fear. It shifts us into our sympathetic, fight, fright, and flee state.

Understand this: every breath you take sends one of two messages to your brain: "I am safe," or "I am not safe." The interpretation of that message globally affects your entire being and expression, breath by breath, moment by moment.

In an effort not to get too deep, I'll just say that mouth breathing not only tells your body to be afraid, but it also invites fear into your body. Constantly living in our sympathetic state, our threat state, ultimately hampers and impairs our thinking. It dials up the sensitivity of our emotions and erodes our emotional intelligence. It makes us hypervigilant over ourselves through a hypnotic inward focus, blinding us to the world and the people around us. It inhibits our ability to live with compassion and contribute to the world because there is always something gnawing on us from the inside; there is always a tension of fear caused by a threat. If our body is always trying to survive some invisible, subconscious threat, it will eventually tire, become inflamed, break down, and age prematurely.

Along with that, due to the inner woven connection of our soul to our body, our mind and emotions will become buried under anxiety, worry, and misery. Mouth breathing will not only keep us from being and expressing our true selves, but it will also keep us from living our best lives. We cannot grow and become when we are in a constant state of fear.

We can only grow and become when we are in a state of peace.

Nasal breathing leads to that state. We were born in this state, without a care in the world. We were born in a growth state, designed to grow and become amazing expressions of peace, love, and tranquility, with a constant glint of joy. When we breathe in our design, we are constantly telling our brain that we are safe and that all is well. This not only frees our bodies from undue stressors, but also our minds and hearts. It makes everything about our lives better, in the smallest of ways. Yes, nasal breathing can ultimately lead us to be "better neighbors" because, in a state of tranquility, we are not consumed by our own thoughts, whether conscious or subconscious. This allows us to express ourselves fully and confidently.

This is weird to think, I know. But what if subconsciously, you were constantly worried about your survival? Is it possible to be concerned about your safety and not know it? Yes. If you live in a constant state of fight or fright, you get used to it; you may not even know it, but your brain knows it. If your brain can take care of walking without you having to think about it, it can attempt to take care of your fear without you having to think about or even be aware of being fearful. Subconsciously, we can be afraid without necessarily knowing it, although our bodies usually send us messages to let us know. Tight neck muscles, sore lower backs, shortness of breath, nervousness, anxiousness - these are all messages and expressions being sent back from the brain. We are just very good at ignoring them or not understanding their meaning. The point is that fear is a sneaky adversary. It can creep in and camp out without us even realizing it's there. And over time, it can wreck us.

What if you could limit fear's access to you by simply breathing through your nose? **You can!** That's your design. You were not designed to be in a perpetual state of fear. You were literally designed for peace and joy - that's your intended default state of being. The way to enter into that state is through your breath.

I should also point out that nasal breathing is also the way to enter into a state of healing. Remember, we cannot grow when we are in fear, and fear is what leads to damage and decay. We grow when we are in a state of peace, and healing is a form of growth and repair. If your body needs healing, if your soul requires healing, you want to, you need to, make sure you are breathing in your design.

Just in case it is needed, here is a checklist of your breathing design:

Get into a comfortable position; it's your choice.

Close your lips and place your tongue on the roof of your mouth. If you are unsure where this position is, just swallow and notice where your tongue goes. That's where it belongs.

Relax your jaw.

Relax your abdominals.

Breathe in through your nose and allow your belly to expand. If you can, allow your sides and lower back to expand as well.

When you feel the urge to release the inspiration, simply let go and exhale through your nose.

Every time you exhale, try to relax more and more.

Simply repeat this process over and over.

If you need parameters, practice this every day for 3 to 10 minutes, 1 to 3 times per day.

Sounds like rocket science, doesn't it? I know it may seem too simple to be useful, but try it. Notice how you feel when you do it. Even just practicing this for three minutes can give you a wonderful sense of peace and well-being. Imagine living this way, breathing this way day in and day out. This is your design. Get familiar with it. Get good at doing it. Breathing in your design leads to life.

Intentional Breathing

Beyond breathing the way we were born to breathe, we can also be intentional with our breath and use it to accomplish various things. From lifting heavier weights to navigating difficult conversations, to meditation, to healing injuries, to emotionally regulating our brains, we can learn to use our breath and our design like a master carpenter uses a hammer — skillfully.

I cannot possibly begin to cover all of the ways that breath has been used throughout the ages to enhance our experiences and explore our existence with ourselves and our Union with all of Creation. However, I can share some of the ways that have been particularly helpful to me in preserving my own life. I hope that you, too, will find some of these very useful.

Getting Ahold of Yourself

"Be angry and do not sin." –EPHESIANS 4:26

That verse could just as easily say, "Be afraid, but do not freak out."

When we get overcome by our negative emotions, we often react through our *less-than-best* selves. Our sympathetic nervous system kicks in with its overstimulating cocktail of adrenaline and cortisol, and we either fight for our opinions or tuck tail and withdraw inwardly from our conversations. We may say or do things that hurt others, we may say or do things that disappoint others, and perhaps we even hurt and disappoint ourselves. You probably know this, but when we react, we lose ourselves. The person we want to be disappears, and our darker side reveals itself, as in the scene where Evil Superman fought Clark Kent in Superman III. If you saw that movie, you know that Clark defeated the Evil Superman.

Remember, life itself is an emergency; it is constantly emerging.

We can do the same thing. We can defeat our "darker side" by intentionally acting with our breath rather than reacting with our emotions. To do this well, we need to do three things:

1) We need to live in our design of breath. This keeps us in our default parasympathetic state. It may be helpful to think of this as our 'Safe, Compassionate State.' This is important because if we are naturally walking around in sympathetic mode, we are already living on the razor's edge of getting lost in our emotions.

2) We need to know who we want to be. Do we want to live our lives in the resilience of kindness or do we want to live our lives in the fragility of fear? Do we want to make the world brighter and better, or do we want to dim it and drag it down with our drowning emotions? If we know who we are and who we want to be, it can anchor us and allow us to withstand the attacks of fear.

3) We need to learn to listen to and be aware of our emotions. At best, our emotions should serve us. At worst, our emotions enslave us. Emotions are informational energy. Yes, they can be expressed to inform those around us about our current state, but they can also reveal our inner state. If we are quick to notice and

receive that information, we can afford ourselves the opportunity to respond to it intentionally. The rub is that it is a choice. And it's often not an easy one.

Remember, life itself is an emergency; it is constantly emerging. We can react to it and lose ourselves, or we can respond to it and preserve ourselves. There will always be stressful situations. There will always be difficult conversations. There will always be tragedies and losses, some far more severe than others. However, we can navigate through these events without getting lost in them, especially if we know who we are or who we aspire to be. One way to navigate life's emergent events is to deliberately use our breath to breathe away the negative emotions and the negative thoughts these events may generate.

If we recognize our emotional stress growing, we can ease its assault by taking long, slow breaths. Something as simple as taking in a long inhale, like 8 to 10 seconds, and then giving an even slower exhale, like 10 to 12 seconds, could be the interruption your brain needs to say, "We are okay. We've got this. Now, let's navigate."

Just one breath.

That may be all you need. If not, you just created enough time and space for another one.

Let your breath be your response to the emergent event and the emergent emotions. Not only will you feel better because you took a long, slow breath - a long, slow breath can make you feel amazing - but you will feel better because you kept yourself, and you don't have to live regretting any reactions you might have made. Shame and guilt only further drive you into a sympathetic state. They bury you and take life from you.

But confidence builds you, increases you, and it can save you and prepare you for the next thing that life throws at you. Confidence comes from successfully navigating through difficult situations. Confidence can also be built through practice.

It is beneficial to practice responding with our breath in small, uncomfortable situations so that we can be better prepared to respond when faced with big, dire situations.

It is also great practice to simply focus on our breath when everything is going well. Getting really familiar with taking long, slow breaths entrains your brain to become masterful at doing it, but also masterful at responding to it. What if you could train your body to efficiently and effectively deal with stress in an instant? You can. All you have to do is be intentional, show up, and practice.

Learning to harness your breath to manage emergencies can change the entire trajectory of your life. It will make everything about you better from the inside out - it will help you protect your heart and mind, allowing you to be your best, selfless self, one that can serve others around you, even those who may be inadvertently trying to harm you. Emotions get the best of most people…

Just try this.

Set aside 5 to 10 minutes and deliberately practice long, slow inhales with even longer and slower exhales. I guarantee that you will feel great if you do this. You're going to feel so good, you may even think about doing it again on another day.

- Sit in a comfortable position (**this is SO important**).
- Place your tongue on the roof of your mouth and close your lips.
- Inhale long and slow, anywhere from 6 to 12 seconds. Feel the air reach its capacity inside your lungs.
- Then begin letting it go by exhaling longer and slower, for 8 to 14 seconds, until your lungs naturally say, "Okay, enough, let's let the air back in."
- Do this for 10 minutes.

Don't overthink this. In the beginning, you may only be able to breathe in for 4 seconds and out for 5 seconds, and that is GREAT! With practice, you will find that you can eventually get to a point where you can easily breathe 4 breaths or less in a minute. If you can get there, you can know how great it feels to breathe like this for five to ten minutes. This is a worthwhile, dedicated practice. If you can do this daily, or almost daily, it can change your life. By the way, the above method is an excellent gateway into meditation and prayer.

Also, try this.

Watch for negative emotions. You can usually spot them quickly, as they usually accompany information that you do not like. Anything that threatens your ego's comfort will elicit internal negative emotional chatter. When you sense it, breathe it away.

Stop. Breathe (long and slow). Repeat.

Use every would-be *less-than-desirable* situation to practice. In each situation, breathe until you can respond in the way that you want to respond. If you feel the surge to react, keep breathing. Your breath is life to you in so many ways.

Being Still

If you were paying attention, you could see that breath can preserve you by calming you. And as I mentioned, it can serve as a gateway to mediation and prayer. When we set aside time to breathe, when we set aside our lives to just sit and breathe, we can discover an unusual stillness.

Original Strength's Pressing RESET system teaches that proper breathing is like a RESET button on our nervous system, and it is. It lets our brain know we are safe, and it optimizes everything about us. But intentional breathing is like a PAUSE button. It also lets our brain know we are safe, bringing a powerful stillness to everything in us, even our thoughts (create stillness), echoing 'Be still and know.'

The two primary messengers of fear are our breath and our thoughts. One of the main reasons we lose ourselves, perhaps the real reason we need to preserve our True Self, is because of our own thoughts. Our thoughts create narrations that enhance and fuel our fears. They are like seeds. If we meditate on them and continually think about them, we nurture them; they grow and take root in our minds, eventually finding a home in our hearts. By the way, this is true for both negative and positive thoughts. The problem is that most people dwell on their negative thoughts. They nurture those negative thoughts, becoming entangled and imprisoned in their roots.

We need to be able to starve our negative thoughts by leaving them alone, by letting them go. This can be approached by learning to have no thoughts, or by learning to let the thoughts that come to us pass by. Both of these approaches are built through practice, similar to strength training. Regular practice can strengthen our ability to let our thoughts happen without grabbing hold of them. It can even help us learn how not to have any particular thoughts. A long time ago, each one of us had this ability. We were once free from thoughts. We were born this way. It was our default state. It can be again, with practice. When we have no thoughts, we have no worries, no stress, no fear, no cares. In other words, we have peace.

Again, you came into this world this way, in peace and with joy. You didn't know how to think, yet a glint of light shone in your eyes, and joy constantly smiled out through your face. There were no thoughts to marinate on, no stories to mull over, no fears to hold your attention. You were purely at peace, and you were joyful (full of joy). This may sound ridiculous, but the state of joy, peace, and love is your natural default state of being.

You can return to this state by suspending the chatter that constantly runs through your mind. You can do this by practicing and focusing on breathing.

One reason this works is that if we focus on our breathing, our breathing has our attention, and our thoughts do not. Another reason this works is that it helps keep us in a parasympathetic state, our peaceful state, which also helps reduce our stress and calm the agitation in our minds. And yet, another reason why this works is that it forces us to withdraw from the world, if only for a little while. It's literally a way to shield ourselves, for a brief moment, from the chaos all around us. It doesn't just help to pause our thoughts; it helps us to pause the world.

Have you ever seen a superhero movie where the hero moves so incredibly fast that the whole world stands still? The hero could see everything he needed to do to save the day, rescue the victims, and defeat the villain. He had peace, clarity, and the ability to respond to everything around him. That's what stillness is like. That's what setting aside intentional time to breathe can do. It slows the world and gives us the opportunity to find clarity, peace, and the ability to respond to emergencies around us.

It also allows us the opportunity to re-experience our True Self—the peaceful, joyful self we were born into. I've said this before in *Be Naked*, but when you experience it, there is nothing that feels better than breathing. What I mean is that if you spend time exploring it, you will come to a place where taking a breath feels almost orgasmic. It can send both amazing energy and peace through your body simultaneously. I know that may be hard to understand, but again, if you find it, you'll know what I'm trying to explain.

Your breath can pause your thoughts. If you can pause your thoughts, you can know peace. If you can learn to pause your thoughts through breathing, you can also learn to pause your thoughts through being, when you are out experiencing the world. Stillness is a great place to practice things we want to do in the absence of stillness. What I mean is that if you can learn to let go and suspend your thoughts when you are still, you can do the same when navigating the challenges life presents.

When you are troubled, when you need to pause the world, get alone, find a quiet place, even if it's a bathroom stall in a restaurant, and practice breathing slowly. Focus on your breath, how it feels, and where it goes. And as best you can, let your thoughts go. If they go, great. If they don't go, great. Just keep breathing nice and slow. It will still benefit you and work for you in some capacity because your breath is life to you.

Breath Prayers

Another breath practice I love to do is using my breath as a prayer. I sit in quiet but wrap specific thoughts, words, or verses inside of my breath.

For example, I may breathe in and mentally say, "I am…" and I may breathe out and mentally say, "…loved by my Father." Done over and over again, I have found this to be quite comforting and peaceful. It helps me cast away the lies of fear or whatever else seems to be attacking me. It also helps me plant positive seed thoughts into my brain. Repeating and rehearsing them with my breath helps these thoughts to take root and flourish.

By practicing this way, I'm combining two sources of "safe" information to my brain: my breath and my words. I am using their combined weight to soothe my soul. This helps me return to my state of peace, love, joy, **and** safety.

You can do this as a prayer, if you like. It can be as simple as

Inhale with "Father," Or "God,"

Exhale with "I need You." Or "I love You." Or "I trust You."

You can also do this as an affirming mantra. It can be as simple as

Inhale with "I can do all things…"

Exhale with "through the Spirit which strengthens me."

Again, this is a powerful way to press PAUSE. It is a way to soothe your soul and preserve your True Self; a way to reveal your True Self, the you that knows peace, comfort, and joy even in the midst of an emergency.

Incidentally, some Jewish scholars and rabbis say that the sound our breath makes is the sound of God's name: YHWH. They say the inhale sounds like "Yah" and the exhale sounds like "Weh." I don't know if this is true, but it is a beautiful thought. I can also tell you that, for me, it feels very peaceful when I practice this. And I can literally feel my body re-

> All of us were born in peace, without any thoughts of fear.

spond to mentally saying these sounds as I inhale and exhale. It's wild. But that could just be me.

What I do know is that the act of breathing is itself a dance with God or a dance with Creation. He fills us with inspiration, and trustingly, we let our breath go to be filled again. We have to exhale to be filled with an inhale. We have to let go to receive. To let go is to trust; there is peace in that. To hold the breath is an act of fear; there is torment in that.

None of us was made for torment. All of us were born in peace, without any thoughts of fear.

Physician, Heal Thyself

"...Can these bones live?" –EZEKIEL 37:3

From what we've discussed so far, it may be easy to see how the breath can be used to help the body and soul heal. However, breath can also be used to help target healing in specific locations of the body. Or, the breath can be used to target specific areas in your body for the pure joy of exploration. Either way, the following breathing method is worth considering.

You can breathe into the areas of your body that you focus on. I know this sounds nuts, but you can learn to do this through practice. You already know this is true. How do you learn or relearn to breathe down into your belly? By focusing on your belly and trying to pull breath there. You can do the same thing in other areas of your body. Some areas are much easier than others, but with practice, you may find that all areas become easy to breathe into, eventually. This can be an essential skill because there may be times when we can help the body heal faster through "breathing into" an injured area.

OK, let's be real, air is not going to go from your lungs into your right butt cheek magically. BUT, you can create the feeling and sensation of your breath reaching your right butt cheek through your directed intention and attention.

You need to set aside a little time and be curious. You can practice and learn a lot in only ten minutes. If this sounds nuts, let's try it. All you have to do is breathe and direct your breath and attention to the areas you are trying to reach. We can start small and then work on finding bigger or more challenging places.

- Get to a quiet place where you can focus.
- Get in a comfortable position.
- Close your lips and your eyes. Don't go to sleep!
- Rest your tongue on the roof of your mouth.
- Set a timer for 10 minutes and begin. When the timer stops, stop (you may not want to!).
- Go only as far as you are successful and/or want to go.
- If you find this, GREAT! If you don't find this, GREAT! We are practicing to learn and grow. It is okay if that takes time.
- Let's start with your nostrils.
  - Focus on your nostrils and feel the sensation of your breath entering your nostrils.
  - Feel the breath go in and feel the breath go out.
  - Stay here and practice this as long as you like. It is quite peaceful.
  - If you've got this, and you're ready, move on to the next part.
- Focus on your sinus cavities, located behind your cheeks, and breathe into them.
  - Can you feel the air entering your cheeks, just below your eyes?
  - Can you feel the air tickling the back of your eyeballs?
  - Stay here and practice this as long as you like. It is very peaceful.
  - If you've got this, and you're ready, move on to the next

part.
- Focus on and breathe into your throat.
  - Can you feel the coldness of the air moving through the middle of your throat?
  - Can you feel your neck expand?
  - Stay here and practice this as long as you like. It is very peaceful.
  - If you've got this, and you're ready, move on to the next part.
- Focus on your right shoulder and breathe into it.
  - Can you feel your shoulder spread as you inhale?
  - Can you feel your shoulder relax and return to its normal position as you exhale?
  - Stay here and practice this as long as you like. It is very peaceful.
  - If you've got this and you're ready, move on to the next part.
- Focus on your left lung and try to isolate your breath in it.
  - Can you feel your left ribcage expand and contract?
  - Can you feel the extra fullness of your left lung as you inhale?
  - Stay here and practice this as long as you like. It is very peaceful.
  - If you've got this, and you're ready, move on to the next part.
- Okay, let's try a harder, yet rewarding, one: focus on your pelvic floor, or the area of your "undercarriage" (this is a family show...), and breathe into that.
  - If you are sitting, can you feel your pelvic floor spread and push against your seat?
  - Can you feel the tension in your pelvis grow with your inhale and shrink with your exhale?
  - Stay here and practice this as long as you like. It is very peaceful and somewhat wild.
  - If you've got this and you're ready, move on and explore any part that you want to breathe into.

For what it is worth, you can help bring healing into an area by bringing your attention and breath to that area. You can even combine the Breath Prayer above with this technique. For example, if your left shoulder hurts, you can breathe into it while you pray for it. Like this:

Inhale into your left shoulder and think, "My shoulder can heal..."

Exhale out of it and think, "...and be made whole again."

This is just an example, but it can be a powerful tool. In doing this, you are combining three powerful elements:

1) You are breathing in your design, telling your brain that you are safe and it's okay to grow and heal. It's harder to heal when your brain thinks you need to shrink to survive.
2) You are planting positive seeds of information into your brain, again sending a powerful message of safety.
3) You are bringing intention and resources, like life-giving oxygen, to that area in need. Before you balk at that, did you feel your shoulder move? Did you feel your pelvic floor move? What moved it? Resources. Blood flow. Intention.

Sometimes we need to heal from pain and injury that aren't physical. Sometimes we hurt in our souls, in our minds, and in our hearts - though this hurt often manifests itself physically. When we hurt on the inside, the body finds ways to express it on the outside. Our bodies are essentially expression suits. Anyway, one of the most wonderful things about using the breath to heal is that it can also help us let go of the hurts we have inside. We talked about this above. We can exhale stress, anxiety, and fears.

You've likely experienced this before. Have you ever made a big sigh of relief and felt your shoulders drop and your neck loosen up? That's because you exhaled tension from your muscles. Tension is nothing more than fear and stress being held within the muscles. When your shoulders dropped from that "sigh of relief," you were letting tension (stress, anxiety, etc) out of your whole being.

If you are hurting on the inside, it can be helpful to imagine that you are inhaling light and love and exhaling fear and pain. It's almost like an imaginative breath prayer. You breathe light into your soul, and then you exhale darkness from it. It may also help to imagine feeling the light, warm energy entering your body. And feel the cold breath of darkness and pain leaving your body. I know it takes imagination, but where the head goes, experienced reality often follows. You may be amazed at how good this can ultimately feel.

Just in case, and it probably doesn't need to be said, but when it comes to healing, we don't want to sow and nurture negative seeds of doubt and fear. Let those go. Don't dwell on them. Don't listen to them. They don't allow healing. In fact, they give you what you think about. We will discuss this further later, but for now, just breathe.

"…Surely I will cause breath to enter into you, and you shall live."
- EZEKIEL 37:5

MOVEMENT PRESERVES

"Engage" —Captain Jean-Luc Picard

I spent a lot of time on breathing because life starts and ends with breath. However, there are other essential means of True Self Preservation.

> Movement also keeps our minds, hearts, and souls healthy.

One of those is moving. I often refer to moving as *living in our design*. I do this because we are clearly designed to move. Movement builds us, grows us, keeps us, and helps to heal us. If we don't live and move in our design, we break down, shrink, get sick, get depressed, and lose ourselves.

Remember, everything affects everything. A healthy body leads to a healthy soul. If we are designed to move to keep our bodies healthy, then movement also keeps our minds, hearts, and souls healthy. Our physicality is not isolated from our mental and emotional well-being. In fact, it's deeply interwoven into them.

Again, our bodies are expression suits. So what are they expressing? They express the "inside" of us.

Whatever is happening on the inside is made known on the outside. This street runs both ways, though; whatever we do on the outside "feeds" and informs our inner selves.

Much of what we do and what we don't do is still boiled down to one question the brain is always asking: "Am I safe?" If we live and move in our design, the answer the brain receives is "YES." That 'yes' makes its way into our subconscious mind and soul through a happy, regulated brain housed in a body that feels amazing because it is doing what it is designed to do.

If we don't move in our design, then the brain doesn't receive all the information that it knows it should be getting. Something (a lot of information) is missing. In the absence of information, in the silence of sedentary living, the brain determines "NOPE, not safe."

That NOPE is taken as a threat, and the brain inhibits various functions, such as range of motion, strength, power, and even digestion and immunity. Living in a state of constant threat day in and day out, in a fight-or-fright mode, stresses the nervous system and, consequently, the body. This stress also seeps into our subconscious, making us anxious, easily agitated, fearful, and stressed.

Is it safe?

When the answer is yes, we can access our True Self. When the answer is 'nope,' we are likely going to require rescue. Just as we remember how we are designed to breathe, we can also recall how we are designed to move. In doing so, we can move towards healing, growth, and self-preservation. In other words, we can find ourselves through movement.

I've written several books about the specific movements we're designed to make to build ourselves into resilient human beings. I'm not necessarily going to dive into those particular movements here. I'm going to approach our movement design from a slightly different angle this time.

Here is what you need to know: Each of us was born with a movement-detection system, known as the vestibular system. The vestibular system also detects gravity. It is designed to detect how we move in relation to the Earth's gravity. It is perhaps one of the most sensitive and brilliantly designed movement detection systems man can even conceive of. The vestibular system, along with some preprogrammed reflexes, is designed for one chief operation, the operation of all operations: Protect the brain.

Every movement you make, and every movement that happens to you, no matter how small, even down to a 0.4° range of motion, is instantly detected through your vestibular system and then sent to your brain. The brain takes that information, assesses it, and then sends a response command down through the body. This all happens before you even realize it.

You've experienced this a million times. Has anyone ever bumped into you on a crowded street? Did you lose your balance and fall? Likely not. Did your body adjust, rotate, stiffen, and right itself to keep you going on your merry way? Did you tell it to do that? Did you even have time to think about it? No. Your vestibular system and its relationship to your brain play a crucial role in maintaining your brain's health and well-being by controlling and adjusting your body's movements. This all happened within milliseconds. As with our superhero movie analogy discussed above, your brain is so fast that it makes time stand still, especially in your conscious awareness.

Your vestibular system is designed to detect movement to help protect AND build your brain. That means your body is also designed to move, providing your vestibular system with information to help your brain develop. What happens if you don't move? You create nothing to detect. Not having information is not only a threat; it can eventually weaken and degrade the vestibular system's ability to detect information. By the way, did you know that every muscle in your body is neurologically connected to your vestibular system? Those connections are designed to be efficient and fast. But like all things in the body, if we don't use them, we weaken them. If we don't move often, as we were clearly built to do, we weaken both our vestibular system and the neural connections that run to and from it.

Worse still, when we don't move often, we weaken the tissues that those neural connections support. Muscles, tendons, cartilage, and bone - all of these atrophy and weaken when we do not move in our design.

I should pause here to note that this is not an endorsement of exercise. Exercise is a band-aid attempting to splint what neglect has done. Exercise can have merit, but exercise won't preserve us, especially if "exercise" is done in the gym with very limited motions in very limited time frames. What I'm talking about is movement - that thing we were born to do, that vehicle of information intended to help us grow and thrive in body, mind, and soul.

Movement keeps us. It strengthens us. It protects us. It enriches our experiences and our existence. It literally nourishes our brain and preserves our entire body's functionality. And, it feeds our souls.

Do you know why there are so many stressed-out, angry, fearful people in the world today? One reason is that we've traded the information our brains were designed to generate and process for the external information of the world. We consume "news," "media," and toxic agendas while being predominantly sedentary. We aren't even using movement to "shake it off" or "walk it off." We are feeding the brain negative information and then focusing on it without even giving ourselves a mechanism to remove it. We are getting lost in the world's emergencies.

Anyway, to heal and grow, we need to do what we were created to do, making the most of our time and experience here in this life. We need to move.

You were designed to show up every single day and move a little and often throughout the day. You are designed to change positions regularly throughout the day. In the following section, I'm going to show you how to easily do this with the movements you were designed to make. All you have to do is show up and engage. If you do that, your body will take care of the rest.

Stop and Give Me 10

Movement heals. Actually, regular movement heals. However, some movements are more powerful than others, especially our foundational movements; they are full of power and potential.

The human body is capable of performing limitless movements and combinations of movements, at least as far as AI is concerned. But no matter how countless and complex the movements are, they are all built on the few foundational movements we were all born to make.

Owning our ability to breathe well, controlling the movements of our eyes and heads, fluidly rolling and rotating, smoothly rocking back and forth, seamlessly transitioning from one position to another, and effortlessly expressing our gait pattern through crawling, walking, or running - these are our foundational movement patterns. When we do these things well, we flood our brain with SAFE information. When we do these things well, we teach our bodies how to move as one whole, poetic movement masterpiece. When we do these things well, we nurture and soothe our souls.

These movements are so powerful, I call them Resets. Engaging in them is like Pressing RESET on your nervous system and body. These movements make everything about you work better; they give you more access to your life by helping you optimize your state of being. In other words, they help you preserve yourself.

Another wonderful thing about these movements is that their results compound. You don't need to do them for hours a day; mere minutes will suffice and soothe your whole body and preserve your well-being. The truth is, if you do them regularly, their roots take hold inside of you. Eventually, as those roots deepen, every movement you make can end up being a RESET. This happens because your foundation of movement supports and infuses all the other movements you make.

Here is my best advice to you and one of my biggest hopes for you: Get acquainted with your foundational movements. Get ridiculously good at doing them. Own them. If you do, they will help to keep you, to preserve you; you'll age well, in strength, health, peace, and joy. Everything affects everything…

Here is a ridiculously simple movement plan to own your foundational Resetting movements. We will practice just one movement for 10 minutes a day. Every day will have a different movement practice and focus.

Here is both the example and the template:

SUNDAY - BREATHE

Practice breathing in your design for 10 minutes. Don't roll your eyes, that's for Monday. Besides, this is going to help you feel amazing for the rest of your life. You can stay in one comfortable position, or you can explore several positions. Your only objective is to practice breathing. You can use any of the methods we mentioned above.

These are the rules:
- Keep your tongue on the roof of your mouth, especially on the inhale. If you are practicing any of the breathing techniques I mentioned in *Be Naked*, such as sighing or counting on exhalations, you can move your tongue as needed. Otherwise, rest the tongue on the roof of your mouth the whole time.
- Try to fill the bottom of your lungs first, or at the same time that you fill the top. Don't overthink this, but do enjoy the experience.
- Make sure your exhalation is at least as long as your inhalation or longer. It's fun to play with a metronome, watch, or breathing app here.
- Notice what you feel and also how you feel. This practice is an opportunity to learn and explore.

MONDAY - LOOK AROUND

Practice controlling the movements of your eyes and head for 10 minutes. This is an excellent opportunity to reintegrate or refresh the movements of your head with your body's neural connections and reflexes. It's also a fantastic way to begin restoring both the eyes' and the neck's range of motion. The better your eyes and neck move, the better your body moves.

You can practice eye and head movements in any position. Because the possibilities are endless, I'm going to funnel you into just a few.

Head Nods while lying on your back in a comfortable position:
- You can place a bolster under your head if needed.....
- Try to look at your sternum, as if you are looking for chocolate ice cream on your shirt.
- Allow your chin to tuck into your throat (as if you were training to make a double chin).
- Raise your head off the floor as if you are trying to look through your feet, but don't lose your chin tuck or your double chins.
- Keep breathing and do not hold your breath.
- Relax your eyes (return them to the ceiling), lower your head, and release the chin tuck.
- That's one repetition.
- Explore these for one to two minutes within your ten-minute session.

Head Rotations while lying on your back in a comfortable position:
- You can place a bolster under your head if needed...
- Slowly rotate your eyes left and right. If you feel fine, incorporate the head rotations below. If you feel dizzy, just explore eye rotations and the range of motion you can move without dizziness.
- If you are not dizzy, rotate your eyes to the right, and then rotate your head to the right. Move as far as your body allows you to go without pain.
- Then, rotate your eyes to the left and rotate your head to the left. Again, only rotate as far as your body allows without moving into pain or dizziness.
- Your head can remain in contact with the floor the entire time. But you can also lift it to rotate it if you want to. Either is okay. Explore both.

- Keep breathing and don't hold your breath.
- Explore these eye and head rotations for a few minutes inside your ten-minute session.

Head Nods on your hands and knees:
- Get on your hands and knees and place your eyes and head on the horizon.
- Moving your eyes and then your head, look to see if there is ketchup on your shirt at your sternum.
- Then, moving your eyes and your head, look up to see if you can see the ceiling.
- Move where your body will let you move. Any movement is GOOD movement.
- Keep breathing. Don't hold your breath.
- Explore these eye and head nods for a few minutes inside your ten-minute session.

Head Rotations while on your hands and knees:
- Get on your hands and knees and place your eyes and head on the horizon.
- While keeping your head level with the horizon, rotate your eyes to the right, then your head to the right.
- You are trying to look over your shoulder as if to see your back pockets.
- Then rotate your eyes to the left, then your head to the left, and look for your left back pocket.
- Keep breathing and don't hold your breath.
- Explore these eye and head rotations for a few minutes inside your ten-minute session.

You can explore eye, head, and neck flexion and extension, as well as eye, head, and neck rotation, in any position. Explore them all. The better range of motion you have with your eyes and neck, the better you can move and the stronger you can be.

TUESDAY - ROLLING

This will likely be your favorite day of the week. If you spend ten minutes exploring all the ways you can roll, you will fall in love with rolling. And, if you roll enough, you will discover a fluidity that feels and looks amazing. I'm letting you know that, because in the beginning, rolling may feel more like a train wreck than a beautiful movement. Just keep exploring it, and eventually your movements will look like poetry in motion.

The other thing you should know about rolling is that it is the beginning of the human gait pattern. Rolling is like walking; it uses both hemispheres of the brain, it connects the opposing limbs, and it teaches the spine how to rotate. When you roll fluidly, you are likely to walk and run very fluidly as well.

Rolling also helps the brain feel very safe, as it tells the brain where everything in the body is located; it creates a movement map for all the body's members and helps solidify their reflexive connections. Again, this may be your favorite day of the week.

Here are some "easier" feel-good rolls:

The Windshield Wiper:
- Lie on your back with your arms perpendicular to your side.
- Pull and bend your knees up towards your chest, so that your feet are in the air and your tailbone is no longer in contact with the floor.
- Gently rotate your legs from side to side.
  - Rotate them as far as you can without your shoulder blades leaving the floor.
  - If your shoulder blades try to leave the floor, hang out in that spot and just breathe, or simply rotate in that range of motion. If you hang out and breathe, you may discover that your brain allows you more range of motion.
- Keep breathing and don't hold your breath.
- This is a fantastic way to restore mobility to your thoracic spine (the area between your ribs) and improve your posture and shoulder mobility.

- You should explore these for several minutes within your ten-minute session.

The Elbow Roll:
- Lie on your belly with your arms overhead, like Superman's flying position.
- Take your right elbow and reach with it as if you are trying to touch the floor behind you.
- Look at your elbow as you reach behind you; this causes your eyes and head to "pull" the body along.
- Allow your body to follow this reach.
- If this feels amazing, you're welcome!
- Then return your eyes, head, and right arm to the starting position.
- Repeat this process with your left elbow, working the two rolls back and forth.
- Keep breathing and don't hold your breath.
- You can also explore these for several minutes within your ten-minute training session.

WEDNESDAY - ROCKING

If the ten-minute rolling session is not your favorite, it's only because the ten minutes of rocking are; Rocking soothes the soul. You already know this, but rocking calms and settles our nerves. It is a movement that takes away the brain's cares and fears. You will likely find that once you rock for ten minutes, you feel pretty amazing in all of you: mind, body, and soul.

Rocking doesn't just soothe the soul, though; it soothes the body through connection. Rocking connects every joint in your body and teaches them all how to work together. It also teaches each joint how it is designed to move by turning on the joint stabilizers, allowing the joint movers to perform their jobs. The body learns how to move and express itself posturally through rocking. It is a gentle movement that can unlock the athlete in all of us.

Here is a fun, explorative ten-minute guide to rocking:

Rocking:
- Begin by getting on your hands and knees.
  - If you don't have a soft floor, get a nice mat or knee pads.
- Place your eyes and head on the horizon.
- Keep your sternum tall and back "flat" (Think Proud Chest or Silverback Gorilla).
- Without dropping your head or rounding your back, push your butt back towards your feet and then rock forward over your hands.
- Simply rock back and forth for a couple of minutes.
  - Keep breathing, don't hold your breath.

Explorative Rocking Ideas:
- Draw circles by imagining your belly button is a magic marker.
  - Work in both directions.
- Draw infinity symbols or write your name in cursive with your belly button as you rock.
- Rock with your eyes closed while listening to waves crash on the seashore.
- Play with different foot positions.
- Play with different knee widths.
- Explore different rocking speeds; rock fast, rock slow.
- Rock while you hum.
- Rock while you smile.
- Rock on your forearms and knees.
- Combine rocking with head nods and head rotations.
- Rock in all the ways your mind and body come up with. If you show up, you'll learn new ways.

THURSDAY - CRAWLING

I'll be honest, I crawl for ten minutes every day. I don't just do this because I know how good it is for my brain and body, I do it because I love it. I can actually feel "strength happening," or being born through this ridiculously gentle movement. I have found that I think really well while crawling; I'm creative and can solve problems. For me, crawling is an opportunity to learn how to move and control my body and my mind. It just makes my day better. By the way, I'm crawling on my hands and knees, not my hands and feet. As I've gotten older, I've learned that the gentle strength found in crawling on my hands and knees gives me access to the strength I want in other areas of my life. I don't have to crawl on my hands and feet for ten minutes to be stronger - I can, and I still love to do that occasionally, but crawling on my hands and knees actually gives me what I want; it makes me feel good.

And believe me, it feels good to feel good.

Crawl like this:
- Get on your hands and knees.
  - If you don't have a soft floor, get knee pads.
- Place your eyes and head on the horizon.
- Keep your sternum tall and back "flat" (Think Proud Chest or Silverback Gorilla).
- Without dropping your head or rounding your back, crawl by moving your opposite limbs together.
  - Feel their natural rhythm.
  - Feel what happens in your body as they leave the floor together and as they return and transfer the weight of your body together.
  - Learn from this experience. Explore it.
- Crawl forward, crawl backward, crawl sideways, crawl in circles.

Explorative Crawling ideas:
- Crawl in super-slow motion. This is where you learn and develop motor control.
- It's also where you learn, develop, and refine stability and mobility.
- Pretend you're an animal and you'll likely move like that animal.
  - Pretend you're a cat.
  - Pretend you're a silverback gorilla.
  - Pretend you're a komodo dragon.
- Crawl with your eyes closed.

- Crawl with exaggerated limb movements (like combining birddogs or fire hydrants with crawling).
- Explore your breathing as you crawl. This is gold!

FRIDAY - SITTING TRANSITIONS

This is a really fun movement session. By exploring all the ways you can transition in and out of sitting, you can learn to move and begin to expand your movement options. The more movement options you have, the healthier and more resilient you are. Exploring sitting transitions is a way to "age-proof" your body and ensure a quality of life, not just a quantity of life. Don't miss this: being able to move well is one of THE keys to a high quality of life.

Spending time learning how to move in and out of positions on the floor fills in your "movement gaps" and further establishes your foundation of reflexive strength, allowing you to have more access to your body's ability to freely express itself. In other words, this helps you feel good and do good in your world.

This movement session is tailored to your personal needs and abilities. We all have different proportions and abilities. Exploring sitting positions reveals where you can and cannot move. It is actually a wonderful way to learn how to move beyond your limitations. If you have restrictions, you don't push through them; you learn from them. Where can you move? How can you make that movement smoother? If you are curious and don't try to force your body into those restrictions, you may find they actually melt away. At the very least, you will learn how to move very well within your body's established parameters.

Because exploring sitting transitions is so person-specific, it would be hard to encapsulate all the different ways to engage in this session. So, please view this video for ideas on how to explore your ability to move in and out of sitting positions.

https://youtu.be/i8DIeiZEtFE?si=ClleXJLpFOeRRV_a

But here are some general guidelines:
- Sit on the floor and explore how you can move in and out of sitting positions.
  - Crawl out of them, roll out of them, lie down from them, stand up from them, etc.
- Play with slow-motion movements.
- Play with different ways to sit.
- Find your limitations and be curious about them.
  - Play and explore for 10 minutes.

SATURDAY - PLAYER'S CHOICE

This is the day when you take ten or twenty minutes and engage in your favorite RESET(S) or movement(s) that you performed earlier in the week. If you absolutely loved rolling and rocking, do them both for ten minutes! This is your day, pick at least one movement and explore it for 10 minutes. Choose the one you want to master, or choose the one that makes you feel the best. Just engage. You'll be glad you did once you've done it.

That's it, that's the simple *ten-minute-a-day* plan for the week. If you do decide to do this, I believe you will discover some wonderful things about your body, but you'll also discover how good it feels to move so well. And that's our design, we are designed to move well and feel good. This is just a simple approach to doing so.

Naturally, depending on your needs, you can do more than this, and you can certainly stack any other physical training you want to do on top of this. These sessions can make a great warm-up or movement prep for your weight training routine, but more importantly, they can help you move better so that your other desired training routines are more effective, more enjoyable, and safer. The return is far greater than the investment. If you have the time and desire, this daily ten-minute movement focus is a fantastic way to learn how to move and set your body free.

Designed to Walk

This is wild to say, but in today's health and fitness world, breathing and walking are the "new" hot thing. It's wild because these are the things humans are designed to do amazingly well (their patterns live in our nervous system), and somehow we've gotten to the point where we have to be told how to do them.

There are several books and teachers out there promoting the benefits of walking. I'm not sure I can add much more to that discussion, though I will reiterate some highlights. What I can bring to the discussion is our design to walk. Walking is the one movement we were clearly made to do. We are the only bipedal mammals in the world, and we are designed to walk efficiently everywhere using our four limbs—the contralateral movement program for walking lives inside our spinal cord. Because we are weak as children and designed to build strength

> We fail to engage in the very things we were created to do.

over time, the pattern begins with crawling or creeping, but as we gain strength, it transforms into walking.

Everything that has a design is designed for a purpose. Anything created, like a hammer for example, that is not used for its purpose will fall short of its glory. A hammer makes a poor screwdriver and a terrible saw. Yet a hammer is perfectly crafted to drive nails. Likewise, we are designed to walk, and walking is the movement intended to maintain and restore our health in mind, body, and soul. However, if we forgo that design and instead spend the majority of our time sedentary, sitting, lying, or standing, we too will fall short of our intended glory. If we don't fully participate in the one thing we were clearly designed to do, our design cannot perform as intended, and we will not be able to fully maintain our health. We will become weak, frail, scared, anxious, demented, withdrawn, and self-consumed.

To say this another way, we were not designed for cars. We designed cars for us. We were not designed for shoes. We designed shoes for us. We were not created for chairs. We created chairs for us. There is nothing wrong with any of these things; we use them for our convenience. The problem comes when we rely on these things or "abuse" them for convenience. When our conveniences remove the need for us to engage in our design, we start living outside of our design - we fail to engage in the very things we were created to do. This is when our health declines across all levels of our being; our emotions become unregulated, our thoughts become negative, and our bodies unravel. As a result, we hurt inside and out, and we just don't feel good. The sad thing is that most of us don't even realize we don't feel good because we've become so used to feeling "blah," or worse.

AND this is WHY we should walk often, every day, throughout the day. It's what we were created to do.

Yes, walking helps you burn calories. Yes, walking helps you digest your food more effectively. And yes, it is good for your heart, blood vessels, joints, brain, nervous system, immune system, bone density, strength, cells, DNA, and everything else. But really, walking is good for the whole of you - it helps to maintain you, and it allows you the opportunity to experience your best self.

When we walk, we soothe our brain, and we gain access to creativity and Inspiration. Many mountains have become molehills, and many problems have been solved during a walk. When we walk, we create an outlet for both our brain and our body to work out their issues. Are you angry? Take a walk. Literally, walk it off. Are you anxious? Go outside and walk. Are you tired and lethargic? Walk your way to having energy. I know this sounds nuts, but it isn't. You know that it takes money to make money. Money is currency, like a current. Energy is a current. And sometimes, it takes energy to make energy, to invigorate yourself. A brisk walk will burn away your fatigue and help you tap into energy that makes you feel really good.

But remember, we are designed to walk with four contralaterally moving limbs, where all four limbs dance together to keep us strong and connected, both inside and outside. We are also designed to walk with our gaze and head level with the horizon, standing tall and strong as our four limbs carry us along. And while all of this is happening, we are designed to breathe in and out through our noses, with our tongues resting on the roof of our mouths, pulling air into the bottom of our lungs. Walking like this is living in our design. When we walk this way, we are carrying ourselves in an open posture, and we are breathing through a restful breathing pattern. Walking in our design lets our brain know we are safe and, in turn, allows us to move well and feel good.

This is super easy to experience. Go for a brisk 10-minute walk and notice what you feel and how you feel. Feel your elevated pulse and your quickened breath. Feel your core muscles working as your shoulders and hips dance together around your rotating spine. Feel your mood lighten. Feel your problems melt away or shrink. And, feel your energy surge. These feelings are life happening in your body. You are literally walking yourself alive to the world.

Embrace your design and walk daily. Even if it is only for ten minutes at a time, try to go for brisk walks two to three times a day, if possible. If you have more time, go for longer leisurely walks. Walking after meals is a fantastic way to RESET your whole being. It's also a great way to help your body digest and wisely allocate the food you just ate.

The point is, walk.

I know you have a job, a family, a commute, and all the other distractions of life. I know the one thing you don't think you have is time. Walk anyway. It's worth it.

Walking is one of the main ways you can preserve and even enhance your life. Remember, you are a walking machine, that's your design. To not embrace your design and live in it would be to fall short of all the glory of life you were meant to experience. You're not a rider, a sitter, a stander, or a lier. You're a walker. And maybe a Texas Ranger…!

Keep Calm and Carry On

While we are on the subject of walking, it is a good time to talk about walking with loads attached to or held by your body, also known as loaded carries. I recently realized that "loaded carries" is somewhat redundant, since if I am carrying something, that something is a load. SO, for the rest of this discussion, I'm just going to say "carries."

Carries are an amazingly simple way to build resilient reflexive strength throughout your body. They make you strong and durable, inside and out. With carries, you are loading your gait pattern with external resistance in the form of weight or friction. Yes, depending on how you load the carries, you are compromising your ability to coordinate four dancing limbs, but you'll return to that pattern after you put the load down. But if you are a purist, there are ways to carry weight without taking your natural gait out of the equation; rucking with a backpack or dragging something while wearing a harness are great examples.

The reason carries are so great for building reflexive strength is that they challenge your body's ability to reflexively maintain its optimal upright position. For example, if I am walking with a fifty-pound weight in my right hand, the weight is trying to laterally flex my spine and pull me down to the right. This forces the left side of my torso to reflexively contract harder to prevent me from being pulled over to the right. The heavier the load, or the farther I walk, the more I challenge my body to maintain my optimal upright posture. The position of the load determines the side of my body that will be reflexively called upon to keep me upright. This is such a fantastic way to target the "core." If I want to work the muscles on the right side of my torso, I would carry a weight on my left side. If I want to work my abs, I would wear a weighted backpack. If I want to work my back muscles, I would hold a weight in my arms (like bearhugging a sandbag).

The load can also be distance. Time under tension strengthens the body. You could carry a lighter weight (like ten pounds in a backpack) for two miles, or you could carry a heavy weight (like a 100-pound sandbag) 100 yards. You could also measure the time it takes you to carry your weight a certain distance. This is one way to track whether you are getting stronger.

For example, if I were to carry a 100-pound sandbag for a prescribed distance, I could keep a log of how long it takes me to carry the sandbag that distance. Every time I show up, I can try to best that time. If I do, I'm progressing.

I could also flip the concept and carry the 100-pound sandbag for a prescribed amount of time. For example, if I wanted to carry a 100-pound sandbag for 10 minutes, I could keep a log of how far I could carry it during that time. If, on the first day, I was able to carry the sandbag 200 yards in ten minutes, and three weeks later I'm able to carry the sandbag 275 yards in ten minutes, I know I have made progress; I'm stronger, both inside and out.

I do keep saying, "inside and out." This is because carries can be mentally gruelling. They are hard yet simple. This is why I love using carries for mental resiliency training. Carries are a simple way to make hard things easy. If you show up enough and carry, you train your brain to do hard tasks, all while you are training your body to do hard tasks - they are the same. But if you carry regularly, the weight gets lighter, the distance gets longer, the clock seems to move faster, and you just become stronger and tougher. It's like adding armor around your body and your mind; you just become more resilient.

Carries can also be an act of forcing your will and your body against an object, like pushing or pulling a sled or a car. This is where the brilliance of your design comes into play; your body knows how to reflexively respond to an object of mass that you are trying to move. For example, if you were to try to push a stalled car out of an intersection, you would not walk up to the car, stand as tall as you can, put your arms out at 90°, and think you'll push that car out of the road. Instinctively, and quite reflexively, your body would lean in at the proper angle and stack your bones on top of each other for optimal leverage and power displacement. You wouldn't think your way through this; you would just do this. Pushing and pulling heavy objects makes your body a walking plank, reflexively. It's a great way to strengthen your core while building your legs and your heart.

There are also carries that run straight through your skeleton, because the mass is centered on you. For example, a balanced weight vest will not pull you in any direction; it is trying to compress your skeleton straight into the ground. While these types of carries don't reflexively challenge your core like the other carries do, they still challenge you, and they do have their benefits. Overhead barbell carries are another great example. They challenge your shoulder and spinal stabilizers while also compressing your skeleton and making your body heavier. They also challenge your ability to breathe down into your belly. This places a huge demand on your nervous system and body. As a result, they strengthen your bones, help build resilient shoulders, improve your ability to breathe under tension, and increase your focus. One does not daydream when one walks with a heavy weight overhead...

So far, I've only been discussing carries while walking. The truth is, you can load any gait pattern. Dragging weight or carrying weight while crawling will help you develop a type of strength you've only dreamed about. It's absolutely brutal and wonderful at the same time. It definitely teaches you that you can not only do hard things, but you can do anything.

I perform some type of carry every day of the week. You should consider doing the same. After all, we are designed to walk and carry things. It is a good practice to participate regularly in the design process.

In the hope that it is useful, here are some of my favorite ways to carry, in no particular order whatsoever:

- Suitcase carries with a kettlebell held in one hand by your side
- Farmers carries with two kettlebells held by your side
- Shoulder carries with a sandbag
- Bearhug carries with a sandbag
- Overhead barbell carries in both hands
- Overhead dumbbell or kettlebell carries in one hand
- A weighted backpack (you don't need more than 25 pounds. 10 pounds is my favorite)
- Crawling while dragging a chain or sled (you're welcome)
- Crawling with a weight vest
- Walking with a sandbag balanced on the head
- Pushing a sled
- Pulling a sled with a TRX-like device is used to drag it backwards
- Dragging a sled with a harness
- Walking with indian one-pound clubs in my hands to make my arms longer (you're welcome)

This is not an exhaustive list, but it should get you started. Do yourself a favor and explore carries a few times a week. If you don't know where to put them, they make a great way to end a strength training session. You won't be disappointed. No one ever got upset because they grew stronger.

Carries are more than just movement; they are resiliency builders, making you resilient. When you are resilient, you are confident and not withdrawn or self-concerned. A confident person is safe enough to save the world around them and dangerous enough to do it.

Do Hard Things

When we challenge ourselves, we grow. Engaging in difficult tasks makes us stronger through adaptation and experience. This is the essence of physical strength training, but it works in all areas of our lives. Lifting heavy things improves our physical strength. Doing things we don't want to do improves our mental tenacity. Engaging in difficult conversations enhances our emotional intelligence and improves our ability to communicate effectively. We are designed to overcome challenges through engagement, persistence, and adaptation. I go into this in great detail in *A Simple Book of Strength.*

One of the best things we can do for ourselves is to seek out and embrace challenges, especially physical challenges. Remember, we are whole beings. If we adapt to uncomfortable, difficult physical challenges, we also strengthen our mind and soul. Nothing about us lives in a vacuum. This is one of the most significant benefits of intentional strength training: its effects bleed into the mind and the soul. This means that mental and emotional resilience can be trained through physical efforts.

But even if this were not so, the benefits of intentional strength training are too great to neglect. Being physically strong and getting stronger makes everything about living life easier. It improves your global physical health and capacity. Your muscles and their ability to move you and allow you to impose your will on the world around you are your insurance plan for a quality of life, along with longevity.

What good is longevity without quality? Longevity without quality leads to a prison in your own body. Not being able to care for yourself, dress yourself, go to the bathroom and clean yourself, walk to your mailbox, get outside and see the sun, listen to the birds, breathe the fresh air, laugh with your grandchildren - this would be hell on earth. For most of us, this is avoidable. For all of us, this is not our design. We are designed for strength AND quality of life. But the road to quality is paved through difficulty. Doing hard things builds strength and helps us navigate life with more ease than we otherwise would.

This is why deliberate strength training is so important, if not necessary. This is why we must choose the path of resistance; it makes us stronger, and it makes life easier.

I've written extensively about reflexive strength training in all of my books. Let's assume, for the rest of this conversation, that we all have our foundation of reflexive strength. Assuming this, I'm going to talk about stacking strength on top of that reflexive strength. Specifically, I'm going to talk about weight training.

My friend and famous strength coach, Dan John, is constantly teaching me. He is the King of simple and practical strength training. His Big 3 for strength training is picking up heavy things from the ground (like a deadlift), pressing weight overhead (like a barbell press), and performing heavy carries. Doing these three things systemically builds amazing strength throughout the body, making day-to-day life so much easier and more enjoyable.

PICK UP HEAVY THINGS FROM THE GROUND

Picking up heavy things from the ground is a challenging way for us to impose our will on an object that does not want to be moved. It requires us to get low to the ground, learn how to grip or hold the object, and push the ground away from our combined center of mass once we have a hold of it.

A barbell deadlift is a fantastic way to train this, but it can also be trained with rocks, stones, sandbags, or dead bodies. Whatever medium you use, it just needs to be heavy enough or awkward enough to make it a challenge. If it is a *doable* challenge, the body will learn, adapt, and grow to the point where it is no longer a challenge. This is undeniable proof of strength. When hard things become easier, you are stronger.

Notice I emphasized "doable." The body needs success, YOU need success. While we can get stronger from performing isometrics (trying to deadlift 2000 pounds or an immovable object), it is hard to quantify that strength, and your desire to persist at isometrics will likely diminish due to the lack of reward. However, when we complete a doable challenge, the accomplishment itself is the reward. It boosts our confidence and releases dopamine in our brains. It feels good to know we are strong. This feel-good feeling also spurs us to continue exploring our strength through practice.

Beyond feeling good, our bodies also learn from successfully performing a challenging task. Success is feedback or information that helps us adapt and learn. The more we have success, the more we can refine our technique and explore the sensations and responses of our bodies.

For example, it's one thing to pull a heavy barbell off the floor successfully. It's another thing to learn how to connect our mind to our muscles and pull the bar up more efficiently. The entire process of showing up to continually challenge ourselves grows us and ultimately makes us stronger.

Learn to pick heavy things up from the ground. This is life-proofing work. You want to have strong legs and a strong back. No matter who you are, one day you're going to have to try to lift something heavy from the ground. You're going to want to pick up your grandchild. You'll want to approach your daily tasks with confidence. More importantly, if you are strong enough to pick up heavy things, you are USEFUL. This is an example of putting your mask on first, then helping someone else with theirs. If you are strong, you can be helpful. In this world, the chances are high that we will come to a time when we need to step in and help someone who is in desperate need of assistance. In a sense, we are not just designed to be strong to enjoy our own lives; we are designed to be strong enough to offer our lives to others in need.

Functional strength is prepared strength, and often it is selfless strength.

This is not a deadlift tutorial. It's a call to action. If you don't know how to deadlift or pick up heavy things, find a coach and do some research. Then engage. If you do know how to deadlift, challenge yourself with it a couple of times a week. Perform one to three challenging sets of 3 to 5 reps.

For example, on Monday, perform three sets of 3 reps with a challenging weight. On Friday, perform 1 set of 5 reps with that same challenging weight. If you are successful both days, consider adding 5-10 pounds the following week. We are looking for a doable challenge that forces our bodies to adapt. Keep a log of your progress so that you can see your strength grow over time.

If you hit an absolute lid, use a deload week or take a break for a week. When you return, start back about 15 to 20 pounds lighter than you ended up and begin building yourself back up from there, adding 5 to 10 pounds every week that you are successful with your lifts.

Or, when you hit your lid on progress, consider taking a 40-day tour with Dan John's *Easy Strength* approach and explore the deadlift every day of the week for varying loads (30% to 80% of your "max") and varying sets that total 10 repetitions per day.

For example, if 315 pounds is your lid for five reps and you just can't do more, with Easy Strength, your week *could* look like this:

Monday @ 30% load = 95 pounds x 10 reps
Tuesday @ 70% load = 225 pounds x 3, 4, 3 reps
Wednesday @ 50% load = 160 pounds x 5, 5 reps
Thursday @ 60% load = 190 x pounds 4, 3, 3 reps
Friday @ 80% to 100% loads = 255 to 315 pounds x 2, 2, 2, 2, 2 reps
Saturday and Sunday = Free days

By the way, if you are checking my math, I'm using the 315 for five reps as the 100% max. I'm well aware this is not an actual 100% max, but I like to leave room for "patient growth." We've got all of our lives to train, why rush the experience and jump in too deep?

Anyway, this is a very conservative approach with loads, but this is roughly what training the deadlift *could* look like. The loads and rep schemes can vary day to day. The main thing is to show up and PRACTICE your lifts, etching them into your nervous system and solidifying access to your strength. Arguably, the Easy Strength approach offers fewer "heavy challenges" in frequency, but it does offer the opportunity to challenge your strength. On the other hand, the Easy Strength approach offers the challenge of discipline and consistency, creating the opportunity to practice and perfect your technique and skills for lifting heavy things from the floor. Growth, through learning and application, is still the result, physically and mentally.

When you finish your tour of *Easy Strength*, you can return to the training scheme above or begin a new cycle of your choosing. You can even cycle through a different form of deadlifts or explore a different tool for deadlifts. For example, you could explore picking up heavy sandbags, rocks, or atlas stones for a few weeks.

The benefit of learning how to pick up different objects is that most objects that are not barbells will ultimately force you to round your back in some way. In life, more often than not, when you bend to pick something up, your back is going to round or move into flexion. You might as well strengthen this pattern and position to further your resiliency. Practicing nothing but back extension when lifting from the floor can set your body up for weakness if it is forced into flexion to maneuver around the object you are trying to lift. If our strength training is truly going to serve us, it needs to equip us to apply our strength outside the weight room. There are no elevated and balanced barbells outside of the weight room.

Along with your barbells, explore picking up hard-to-maneuver objects. Make it a practice to build your strength by owning your ability to pick up heavy things from the ground. Life is going to force your hand with this one day, if not every day. You should be skilled at it and confident in your ability to do it. Picking heavy things up from the ground is life-proofing and quality-of-life-enhancing.

PRESS WEIGHT OVERHEAD

When I was a teenager, I lived to bench press. Mostly because my best friend, Patrick Tyndall, told me that girls liked guys with big chests, and that the way to get one was to bench press. Naturally, from that moment on, every day was bench day. It worked, my chest became huge - but it probably looked like I was riding around on a chicken. I did nothing for my legs.

Anyway, as cool as the bench press is, it's not the king of presses; that title is reserved for the overhead press (and its variations). If your shoulder mobility allows, the overhead press is a fantastic strength movement. It teaches your whole body how to contract to move the weight overhead, and it loads your entire skeleton as the weight tries to compress your body into the ground. This makes the overhead press an excellent movement for building muscle and strengthening bones.

The overhead press is also a very functional movement, one that life will likely demand from you quite often. Very rarely will life ask you to lie on your back and press something heavy off your body. But it will ask you to lift or hold something over your head, and when it does, you'll want to be able to do so.

I am a fan of practicing the overhead press a few times a week. This can be done with a barbell, dumbbells, kettlebells, or even through handstand pushups. Ultimately, the barbell lets you explore pressing more weight, but dumbbells and kettlebells let you explore pressing with one arm at a time. There is value in all of it.

Whatever route you choose, consider one to two "heavier" days and one "lighter" day of overhead pressing. On your heavier days, if using a barbell, aim to achieve three sets of 5 reps. On your lighter day, maybe you try single-arm overhead presses for three sets of 8-12 reps.

With the barbell, if you complete all your reps in all your sets, consider increasing your weight by 1 to 5 pounds the following week.

If you are successful in hitting 12 reps in all your sets with each arm on your lighter day, consider jumping up a dumbbell or kettlebell size (depending on your resources). If this jump is too much, either add reps to your set or explore moving more slowly through your reps (make it harder).

IF you are performing handstand pushups, try to work up to three to five sets of 10 reps. When this is doable, consider increasing reps or doing deficit handstand pushups. Deficit handstand pushups are when you place your hands on a bolster (like yoga blocks or small stools) to lower your head below the level of your hands, increasing your pressing range of motion. This builds STRENGTH!

Here are some examples of what this training week could look like:

Monday:
Barbell Overhead Press with 135 pounds x 3 sets of 5 reps

Or Handstand Pushups x 5 sets of 10.

Wednesday:
Standing Kettlebell Press with a 24K (53 pounds) x 3 sets of 10 reps with each arm.

Friday:
Barbell Overhead Press with 135 pounds x 3 sets of 5 reps

Or Handstand Pushups for five sets of 10.

When you hit all your numbers, you could increase the difficulty the following week. When you hit your lid on progress, you could consider taking that 40-day tour with Dan John's *Easy Strength*. Just show up 5 days a week and vary your loads (30% to 80% of your "max"), along with your sets, so that each day totals 10 repetitions.

For example, if 155 pounds is your lid for five reps and you just can't do more, with *Easy Strength*, your week *could* look like this:

Monday @ 70% load = 110 pounds x 3, 4, 3 reps
Tuesday @ 50% load = 80 pounds x 5, 5 reps
Wednesday @ 60% load = 90 x pounds 4, 3, 3 reps
Thursday @ 30% load = 45 pounds x 10 reps
Friday @ 80% to 100% loads = 125 to 155 pounds x 2, 2, 2, 2, 2 reps
Saturday and Sunday = Free days

Again, this is a very conservative approach to loads, but it will work to build and reveal your strength by optimizing your neural efficiency. It also allows you to truly focus on the movements and learn from them. And it will make you naturally curious, as you will find yourself adjusting your percentages and exploring loads beyond your "max" as the weeks go by.

After the 40-day tour of *Easy Strength*, you can return to the previous plan above or explore another set and reps scheme - have fun challenging yourself to grow and learn.

HEAVY CARRIES

I wrote extensively about carries above. Just remember, you were made to carry things. This is one of those things you were just born to do: Pick something up and carry it from here to there. When we carry heavy things that are external to our bodies, our center of gravity changes and moves towards the object we are carrying. This forces our bodies to reflexively respond so that the load we are carrying doesn't pull us out of balance or force us to the ground.

Here is an example I did not use above, but if I'm carrying a 50-pound sandbag on my head, my center of gravity moves from my navel up towards my sternum. This reflexively forces the muscles around my thoracic area to push up against the object. This also causes my center (core) muscles to stiffen and brace my spine much harder than they otherwise would. Walking for any length of time or distance like this will strengthen my entire torso.

Again, carrying heavy loads builds tremendous core strength and stability (as does picking heavy things off the ground and pressing things overhead). But when we carry, we provide the body with opportunities to reflexively endure the strain of resisting the shift in our center of gravity. This reflexive endurance increases our resilience.

When you get good at carrying things for long distances, it means you are stronger. You have carried yourself to the place where what once was hard is not only doable but easy. You have learned to make hard things easy.

That is the secret to carries: To get the biggest bang for your buck, make them uncomfortable. Then show up often until they become comfortable. If you do that, you'll be as strong as you want to be. It's as simple as that.

PUTTING IT TOGETHER

Picking heavy things up from the ground, pressing heavy weights overhead, and carrying heavy objects - these three things can be trained together in a single session, or they can be done on their own. What matters most is showing up and doing them.

Here is a simple template of what combining all three could look like:

Monday:
Warm-up x 10 minutes (this can be any of the 10-minute sessions I listed above)

Overhead Press x 3 sets of 5
Deadlift x 3 sets of 3
Heavy Shoulder Carries x 10 minutes (shoulder a sandbag and walk for 20 yards, switch shoulders and repeat till time expires)

Wednesday:
Warm-up x 10 minutes (this can be any of the 10-minute sessions I listed above)

Kettlebell Press x 3 sets of 10R/10L
Sandbag or Rock Lifts from the ground x 3 sets of 8
Ruck with a 25-pound pack x 30 minutes

Friday:
Warm-up x 10 minutes (this can be any of the 10-minute sessions I listed above)

Overhead Press x 3 sets of 5
Deadlift x 1 set of 5
Heavy Bearhug Carries x 10 minutes (bear hug a heavy rock, sandbag, or ball, walk for 20 yards. Put it down, shake it out, and repeat until time expires)

You could also combine all of this in an Easy Strength fashion. You would simply vary your weight and rep schemes for the lifts and even the carries. You could also just perform a different type of carry every day that you train.

Here is an example of what this might look like:

Monday
Deadlift at 70% load x 3, 4, 3 reps
Overhead Press at 30% load x 10 reps
Suitcase Carry x 10 minutes
- putting the weight down and switching hands every 40 yards for 10 minutes.

Tuesday
Deadlift at 50% load x 5, 5 reps
Overhead Press at 50% load x 5, 5 reps
Rack Walks x 10 minutes
- with a kettlebell or dumbbell in the rack position, walk 20 yards. Put the bell down, switch hands, and repeat for 10 minutes.

Wednesday
Deadlift at 30% load x 10 reps
Overhead Press at 70% load x 3, 4, 3 reps
Sandbag Shoulder Carries x 15 minutes
- with a "heavy" sandbag. Pick it up from the ground, shoulder it, and walk for 20 yards. Put it down, shoulder it on the other shoulder, and walk back. Put the bag down every 20 yards for 15 minutes. (More deadlift practice.)

Thursday
Deadlift at 60% load x 5, 3, 2 reps
Overhead Press at 40% load x 6, 4 reps
Farmers Carries x 10 minutes
- grab two bells and go for a walk. Put them down when you have to. Pick them back up and continue when you recover. Do this for 10 minutes.

Friday

Deadlift at 80% to 100% loads x 2, 2, 2, 2, 2 reps
Overhead Press at 90% load x 2, 2, 2, 2, 2 reps
Ruck x 20 minutes
- with 15 pounds in a backpack - walk with purpose!

Saturday and Sunday
Rest, Play, Explore, Hike, Ride, Swim, Golf, Throw, Catch, etc...

These are just examples. The point is, add more strength to your reflexive strength by doing hard things. If you do hard things often enough, the hard things become easier. This is the evidence of strength growing and working itself out. From a simple strength-training perspective, doing hard things could involve picking up heavy objects, pressing them overhead (or pushing them away from your body), and carrying heavy or awkward objects for a set distance or time. These are great ways to work out your strength.

THE ROOT OF YOUR STRENGTH

While we are talking about building strength on top of reflexive strength, I am compelled to circle back to the importance of having a solid foundation of reflexive strength. Without it, trying to build strength in your body through strength training is like trying to build a house on shifting sand. You'll never be as strong as you were meant to be, and your efforts could end up causing you pain and injury.

This is where the pelvic floor comes in; it is the literal foundation, or the root, of your reflexive strength. It is also the one area of our bodies that none of us wants to think about, talk about, or even acknowledge its importance. But it is crucial, as anyone with pelvic floor dysfunction can tell you. In fact, it is the floor of your core.

The symptoms of pelvic floor dysfunction vary, but commonly include urinary issues like frequency, urgency, leakage, and difficulty emptying the bladder; bowel problems such as constipation, straining, and fecal incontinence; and pain in the pelvic area, lower back, and genitals, often with a full or bulging sensation in the rectum. Painful intercourse and pelvic pressure are also common.

It is estimated that roughly 30% of all people have some type of pelvic floor dysfunction. The numbers are likely higher than this because many people with pelvic floor dysfunction will actually suffer in silence and not seek help, meaning they don't report their issue. The 30% comes from those who seek help. Having said that, even if you do not have a pelvic floor issue, this could be the most important chapter in this entire book. Actually, I'm going to be more direct: **This is the most important chapter in this book. DO NOT SKIP IT.**

I share this PSA because in the courses I teach, I've seen the biggest smiles, greatest movement miracles, and the largest glints of hope during the Pelvic Floor Reset portion. What started as something I dreaded teaching has now become my favorite thing to teach. This information is simply life-changing. If you have a pelvic floor issue, it could help you heal. If you don't have a pelvic floor issue, it could make you stronger by further establishing your reflexive strength through releasing any physical limitations your brain is implementing to protect you.

Having said that, I'm not going to focus on pelvic floor dysfunction. If you do have issues with your pelvic floor, do seek professional medical help; don't suffer in silence. (Yes, this is actually self-preservation, like putting on your own oxygen mask.) But along with seeking help, do also consider the information presented here. What I am going to focus on is the pelvic floor's health and its relationship to the diaphragm. If you can implement this in your life, you will feel better and move better.

I find it fascinating that in Eastern medicine and religion, the pelvic floor is the location of the Root Chakra, the Chakra correlated with security and stability. Remember, the brain is always asking one question: "Am I safe?" In a sense, the answer to the question, "Am I safe?" is expressed, or experienced, in the pelvic floor. Also, remember, the chief messenger to this question is the diaphragm. How we breathe tells the brain whether or not we are safe. This is important because the diaphragm has a "twin," the pelvic floor.

Yes, your diaphragm is intimately connected to your pelvic floor. They are actually twin diaphragms that dance and move together with inhalation and exhalation. In fact, before you even inhale, your pelvic floor and your transverse abdominal muscles both receive electrical signals to prepare them to move with the incoming breath and the movement of the diaphragm. This is why it is so important to breathe into our design. If we are using our diaphragm properly, we are likely employing our pelvic floor muscles as well. In other words, if our diaphragm is dysfunctional, our pelvic floor may very well be dysfunctional. Conversely, if our diaphragm is strong and functioning optimally, our pelvic floor is likely functioning optimally as well.

AND, since these two diaphragms are "twins", they are meant to dance together. If we can strengthen our diaphragm, we should be able to strengthen our pelvic floor muscles. And we can - that's actually how it works, and that's actually how you built a strong pelvic floor as a child, you strengthened and challenged your diaphragm appropriately through growing, developing, and moving.

What I'm telling you is that we can strengthen the floor of our core through targeting our diaphragm through practicing specific breathing techniques, positions, and movements. Before we dive into this, let's discuss "reflexive" strength.

Breathing, though it can be controlled continuously for a little while, is an automatic reflex. Your diaphragm is a muscle that doesn't really tire, nor can it afford to. It moves reflexively throughout your entire life. This means that your pelvic floor, the twin diaphragm of your breathing diaphragm, the one that receives electrical impulses to move with inhalation and exhalation, is also reflexive by nature. Your entire inner core is reflexive - that is the secret and source of your strength.

Reflexive strength is not cognitive strength, nor can it be. If these muscles depended on our cognitive effort to fire, the moment we forget to use them consciously, we could injure ourselves. Cognitive muscles are moving muscles. Reflexive muscles are stabilizing muscles. Our inner core muscles are stabilizers (diaphragm, pelvic floor, transverse abdominus); they hold us and protect us. Stabilizers cannot be cognitive; they must be automatic and reflexive. When our stabilizers are reflexively functioning properly, they tell our brain that we are safe. When we are safe, we are strong and capable.

I'm bringing all of this up because cognitive efforts are traditionally employed to strengthen the pelvic floor muscles. These efforts are called Kegels - the cognitive contracting and releasing of the pelvic floor muscles. I'm not saying Kegels don't have their place, but I am asking: "Should we try to strengthen non-cognitive, reflexive muscles through cognitive contractile efforts?" Or, perhaps a better question is "Should we treat stabilizers like movers in order to make them stronger?"

Stabilizers are reflexive. Your rotator cuffs are reflexive; you do not cognitively try to contract them before you move your shoulder. They fire on their own and should actually fire before your arm moves.

A better example may be your posture.

Your posture is reflexive, an automatic expression of the stabilizing muscles of your body. This is why cognitive efforts to "hold" your posture DO NOT WORK. When we "hold" our posture a certain way, we are using "movers" to become "holders," cognitive muscles to do the job of non-cognitive muscles. The problem is that when they are working properly, non-cognitive, stabilizing muscles do not tire; they reflexively endure. But movers tire; they need energy, and they run out of it when they are being overworked. Movers also take mental energy when they are consciously moved or "held." The moment the brain tires of the effort or forgets to be conscious of the position(s), the movers relax and let go. Thus, posture cannot be held through your willpower. That is not the body's design.

Likewise, the strengthening methods that increase the strength of cognitive movers don't really work for non-cognitive stabilizers. For example, if I want to strengthen my biceps, I may need to do curls or chin-ups - these are movements that employ and challenge the biceps. Kegels are cognitive movements often used to strengthen the pelvic floor, which is composed mainly of reflexive muscles. Pelvic floor dysfunction is often the result of reflexive, stabilizing issues, not a lack of cognitive effort or contractile strength. It is good and great to be able to consciously hold your bowels in a potty emergency, but they should also be held subconsciously and automatically when they are functioning properly.

What I am trying to say is that our pelvic floor should be reflexively strong and "hold" us without our conscious effort. We did not strengthen it consciously as children; we strengthened it through living and moving in our design. I believe this remains the best approach for restoring pelvic floor health and function.

In other words, we need to get great at breathing, exploring our breath, and moving if we want to optimize the health of our pelvic floor. And really, becoming a "master breather" will optimize everything about our lives, especially our pelvic floor.

Ok, now that I've laid the *foundation*, let's explore how to strengthen our floor through breath exploration, positioning, and movement. I encourage you to explore these "exercises" daily. I also encourage you to test them out. Perform a movement baseline, such as a toe touch, squat, or shoulder flexion. Then perform these exercises, retest or check in with your movement baseline, and discover how much easier, smoother, and better your body moves. Test your baseline after each one of these exercises to discover the ones your body really loves. The better you are at moving, the safer your brain feels - the more it loves what you just did. When you find the exercises your brain loves the most, do those often, if not daily.

These exercises will make a massive difference in your life - how you move, how you feel, how you think. Don't trust me, discover this for yourself. And just in case, I'll also leave the YouTube videos I've made with these exercises. It may be helpful to see and hear what's happening, but more importantly, it may be helpful and hopeful to read the comments of the users who have engaged in these exercises. All I can say is that the body is made to heal, and it can...

Ok, I'm going to present the following exercises in phases and steps that mimic our developmental phases as children. You can try them all, but remember to focus on the ones your body loves and feels safe with. Depending on the condition of your pelvic floor, you may overreach. You could not overreach as a child; you had to build the strength to enter into each phase. You can overreach as an adult because you already have the strength that allows you to reach too far. For example, you can already walk, so you may want to start with phase 3. But just because you can already walk doesn't mean your body is actually ready to start at phase 3. Honor where you are, be patient, and allow time and repetition to be your true friends. This is how you developed as a child. If you don't truly know where you are, test these exercises against your baseline and let your body teach you.

Phase 1 - On your back, knees tucked, chin tucked, neck flexed. Keep your tongue on the roof of your mouth unless told to do otherwise.

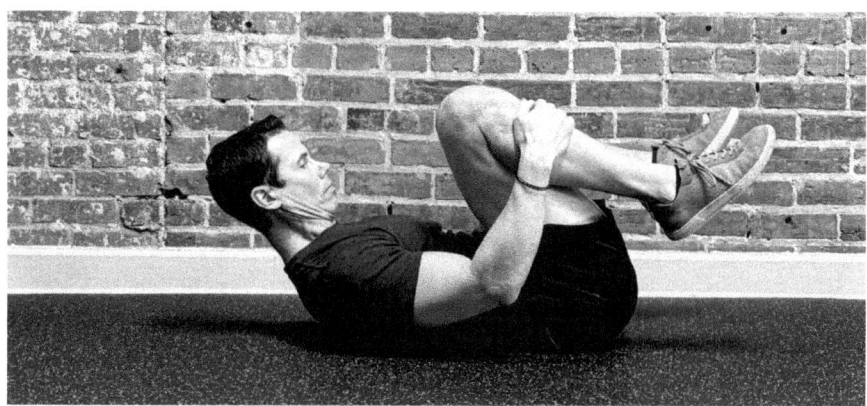

Step 1 - Belly breathe in this position. This may be difficult because this position reflexively contracts the muscles of the anterior chain. By learning to breathe here, we are learning to breathe under reflexive tension - we are challenging our diaphragm and making it stronger. If we are challenging our diaphragm, we are also challenging its twin, the muscles of the pelvic floor. Breathing in this position "turns the volume up" on the diaphragm and pelvic floor, creating more expression or output. As you breathe in this position, notice what you feel. Can you feel your pelvic floor move as you inhale and exhale? It dances with your diaphragm.

Step 2 - Rapidly sniff air into your nose in this position (sniff in quickly and relax just long enough for the air to exit your nose before you rapidly sniff in again). It sounds like this: "sniff, sniff, sniff, sniff, sniff, sniff,

sniff…" If you do this correctly, you will feel your diaphragm and pelvic floor powerfully bounce with the inhalations of the sniffs and rebound down with the relaxations of the exhales. Notice what you feel. Can you feel the powerful movements of your diaphragm and pelvic floor?

Step 3 - Rapidly exhale small bursts of air out of your nose through contracting your abs as if someone were going to punch you (make the "hmmmph" sound and relax). When you squeeze or rapidly exhale with the "hmmmph," your diaphragm and pelvic floor muscles ascend rapidly, forcing some air out of your lungs. When you quickly relax and let go, the air comes back into your lungs. It sounds like this, "hmmmph, hmmmph, hmmmph, hmmmph, hmmmph, hmmmph…" If you do this correctly, you will feel your diaphragm and pelvic floor powerfully jump with the exhalation of the "hmmmphs" and rebound with the small, relaxed inhalation. Notice what you feel. Can you feel the two twins jumping together? Can you also feel your transverse abdominal muscles (your muscle girdle around your midsection) squeezing to assist the diaphragm and pelvic floor muscles? Remember, these three core muscles are always dancing together. They are designed to be a packaged deal.

Step 4 - Mini rocks back and forth. In this same position, rapidly rock back and forth in small ranges of motion (the video ahead may be very helpful here). Keep breathing and do not hold your breath! If you do this right, you will feel that your body actually tries to breathe with the rocking motion. You can also feel your pelvic floor muscles reflexively contract with the rapid change of direction as you rock. Rocking back and forth rapidly spreads the floor of the pelvis, stretching and contracting the pelvic floor muscles. This is another way to strengthen these muscles through playful, exploratory movements, just like you did as a child. Notice what you feel. Do you feel the bounce in your pelvic floor? Do you feel the bounce in your throat? Your vocal cords are another diaphragm that is also connected to your pelvic floor. The human body is amazing, right?

How to Strengthen the Pelvic Floor - Phase 1
https://youtu.be/mxir1-jRsKo

Phase 2 - on your forearms and knees (hands and knees also work if you cannot get here). This is essentially the same position, flipped right-side up. Gravity is the new variable or load.

Keep your tongue on the roof of your mouth unless told to do otherwise.

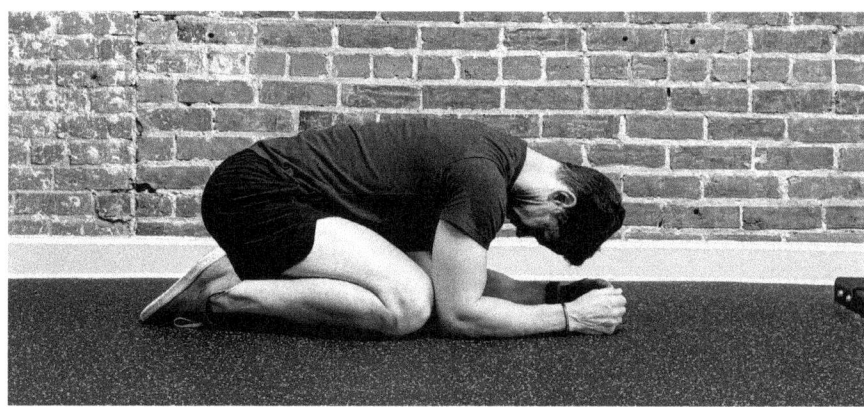

Step 1 - Belly Breathe in this position. This may actually be easier than Step 1 in Phase 1. By learning to breathe here, we are learning to breathe under the reflexive tension caused by the position. Again, breathing in this position "turns the volume up" on the diaphragm and pelvic floor, creating more expression or output. As you breathe in this position, notice what you feel. Can you feel your pelvic floor move as you inhale and exhale? The sensation may be much stronger in this position.

Step 2 - Rapidly sniff air into your nose in this position, just like you did in Phase 1. "Sniff, sniff, sniff, sniff, sniff, sniff, sniff..." If you do this correctly, you will feel your diaphragm and pelvic floor powerfully bounce with the inhalations of the sniffs and rebound down with the relaxations of the exhales. This sensation is likely way more pronounced in this position. Notice what you feel. Can you feel the powerful movements of your diaphragm and pelvic floor now?

Step 3 - Rapidly exhale small bursts of air out of your nose through contracting your abs as if someone were going to punch you (make the "hmmmph" sound and relax). "Hmmmph, hmmmph, hmmmph, hmmmph, hmmmph, hmmmph..." If you do this correctly, you will feel your diaphragm and pelvic floor powerfully jump with the exhalation of the "hmmmphs" and rebound with the small, relaxed inhalation. Again, this sensation may be much more noticeable in this position. Notice what you feel. Can you feel the two twins jumping together with your transverse abdominal muscles?

Phase 2.5 - on your hands and knees. Slightly shift your weight over your hands. Gravity is no longer a load (you'll feel it).

Keep your tongue on the roof of your mouth unless told to do otherwise.

Steps 1, 2, and 3 are the same as above. You can explore them again here.

Step 4 - Hummmmmm. Inhale and exhale by humming all the air out of your lungs that you can. You are going to hum until there is nothing left to hum. As you do this, you will feel your diaphragm, transverse abdominal muscles, and pelvic floor muscles all contract and rise to expel air from your lungs. The more air that leaves your lungs, the tighter and higher they will rise. When you've squeezed all the hum out, LET GO. The air will rush back into your lungs forcefully because your pelvic floor, TVA, and diaphragm will all return to their resting positions. You will most certainly notice this! This is an excellent way to strengthen your inner core and restore your pelvic floor. As you hum all the air out of your lungs, you can keep your lips shut and rest your tongue on the roof of your mouth. This one is fun to practice. It calms and soothes you while it strengthens you.

Step 5 - Mini rocks back and forth. In this same position, rapidly rock back and forth in small ranges of motion. Keep breathing and do not hold your breath! You will feel your pelvic floor muscles reflexively contract with the rapid change of direction as you rock back and forth. Again, this motion and change of direction rapidly spread the floor of the pelvis, stretching and contracting the pelvic floor muscles. For more fun, you can also hum while you do this (just like a child would). I dare you not to smile as you do this. You'll likely notice that you want to. Do you feel the bounce in your pelvic floor? Do you feel like smiling?

How to Strengthen the Pelvic Floor - Phase 2
https://youtu.be/t0zhnQZasSg

Phase 3 - Sit in the squat. If you need to hold onto something to do this, that is okay. We are trying to get back to the same two positions we started, just right-side up this time. Gravity is now different in this same position.

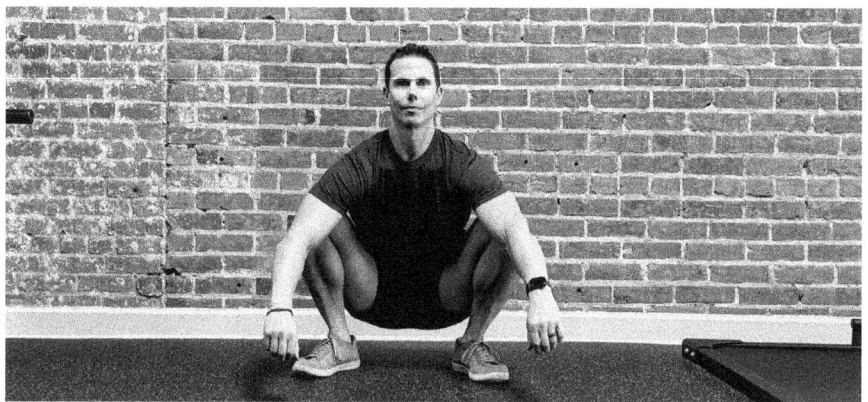

Steps 1, 2, 3, and 4 are the same as above. You can explore them again here. The position and the effect of gravity in this position create new demands on the diaphragm and pelvic floor. Again, we are "turning up the volume" on their expression through challenging them with the resistance position and gravity. Notice what you feel. Can you feel your pelvic floor dance with your diaphragm in this new position with these steps?

Step 5 - Rotate in the squat. Leading with your eyes and head, look over your shoulder and rotate your body as if you were looking behind you. Let your legs naturally follow this rotation. You will notice that the trailing leg will internally rotate and travel down to the floor as the lead leg externally rotates. We are now twisting the floor of the pelvis, applying a new form of stress and tension to the pelvic floor - this strengthens these muscles, especially if we can maintain our ability to breathe as we do this.

Step 6 - Bounce. We can now bounce in small motions while sitting in the bottom of the squat. This is much like the mini rocking we performed on our back in Phase 1 and on our hands and Knees in Phase 2.5. Again, through this bouncing motion, we are rapidly spreading the floor of the pelvis, stretching and contracting the pelvic floor muscles. For extra fun, we can hum here too. Regardless of whether or not you hum, notice what you feel. Can you feel your pelvic floor stretching and contracting?

How to Strengthen the Pelvic Floor - Phase 3
https://youtu.be/eszNHPULvKA

REMEMBER - start where you need to start. You spent years building a strong pelvic floor as a child; it is okay if it takes months to rebuild one as an adult. The body can heal if we honor it and engage in its design for strength. Many of you reading this DO NOT NEED TO START at Phase 3. Phases 1 and 2 are perfect for you. I actually do Phases 1 and 2 every single day because I like how they feel and I know what they are doing for my body; they are making me stronger from the inside out.

Also, the first time you engage in these phases and steps, remember to test a movement baseline to see where you need to be. If your movements continue to improve, awesome! You're doing things your brain loves. If your movements regress or get worse, you've overreached. Take a step back and play with the preceding phases and steps that your brain loves. And remember, if your pelvic floor needs to heal, be patient. Oak trees don't grow overnight. They grow consistently over time. The body heals in much the same way. Healing can start instantly, but its roots must deepen and broaden over time to take effect. Engagement and time are your friends. They are also the way you spent the first few years of your life growing. By the way, another name for healing is growing.

As I said above, and I know this is probably way too much to ask you to believe, but this could be the most important section in this whole book. I encourage you to explore it for yourself. I've seen miracles happen with these movements. I've read of amazing miracles in the comments of the videos associated with these movements. If you can heal or strengthen your pelvic floor, if you can explore your design for breath, you can establish a reflexive floor of safety and stability - while simultaneously reinforcing the message "I am safe" to your brain.

This is the essence of health and strength - living, being, resting, and trusting in our design. This is what you did as a child. This is how you can restore and preserve yourself as an adult. But just in case you didn't notice, the root of all of this goes back to how we breathe. If you could be great at one thing, make sure you breathe well.

EAT LIKE YOU ACTUALLY LOVE YOURSELF

Let's talk about nutrition and how it relates to self-preservation. Food and water are gifts; they provide the nutrients we need to live and express ourselves. Just as we are designed to move and grow from specific foundational movements, we are designed to eat and grow from foundational foods and nutrients.

The point is, there is a design for your body to eat and process gifts supplied by the world. You may call these gifts "whole foods," but they are gifts nonetheless, made for your body. AND, and this is important, your body is made for these gifts. Your body KNOWS how to digest and utilize whole food that comes from the earth. You could even look at food as information - all information that enters your body is interpreted as "safe" or "not safe."

Before we get too deep here, let's address our individuality, our different cultures, our different geographical locations, and our different preferences - we may not all be designed to eat the same foods. Our bodies don't feel safe with all the "information" known as "whole foods." Your body may feel very threatened by strawberries, shrimp, or wheat. If you know your body interprets a food as a threat, that's very useful information, and it should be heeded.

You also likely have beliefs about foods - whether we should eat plants, meat, both, none, or whatever. Those beliefs you hold are also information that ultimately ends up being interpreted as "safe" or "not safe." Therefore, I will not be asking you to violate your beliefs about nutrition or what you should eat. You do *you* the best you can.

Whatever your beliefs, allergies, culture, or seasonal food availability, you still can't get around your design for food and water. You are made to take in proteins, fats, carbohydrates, and water. These are the "rocks" your body's health is built upon. They are all essential to your ultimate well-being. Ideally, we should consume them as close to how the earth presented them to us. I'm not saying we shouldn't process them by cooking or preparing them; I'm saying we probably shouldn't adulterate them with chemicals and man-made concoctions that someone has deemed *Generally Recognized as Safe.*

After all, *Generally Recognized as Safe* could also be seen as "We don't think this will kill you or cause immediate harm in small doses." When it comes to GRAS, would you bet your ass? Sorry, I had to...

Anyway, man tends to try to outsmart his design, and the realm of nutrition and food is certainly no exception. It is where man's cleverness abounds. To be fair, we've created and discovered many wonderful things like food science, the art of cooking, the art of combining foods for flavor and sustenance, and the many ways of supplying nutrition to the sick in hospitals. But we've also created something else - nutrient-deprived, super-convenient, super-easy to consume "food" that sabotages the body's signaling system and hijacks the body's digestive design. Yes, you could look at these foods as ultra-processed, but honestly, unless you're eating your food straight off the vine, tree, or hoof, all food is processed. It's a spectrum. And in case you didn't know, life happens in the middle of most spectrums; we often thrive somewhere in the middle. The extremes are just that - extreme. Extremes lend themselves to survival, compensation, and sickness.

Besides, the processing isn't as much the problem as the sensory hijacking and the Frankenstein nutrition is. Chemicals that preserve, color, sweeten, stabilize, and addict us to food are the problem. So are unstable, over-processed, non-natural fats. Again, we are made to consume macros (carbs, proteins, fats) and nutrients (vitamins and minerals) as close as we can to how nature presents them.

If you live in a first-world country, this can be challenging. Most of your hunting and gathering is probably done in a non-seasonal grocery store - hopefully. If most of your hunting and gathering is done at a fast-food restaurant, not only are you possibly sabotaging your body, but you could also be sabotaging your finances and hindering your ability to buy some really good, nutritious food.

To be a skilled hunter/gatherer in your local grocery store, shop the outside or the edges of the store. Only go in the middle of the store when you need to find things like good monounsaturated or saturated oils, vinegars, or honey. To be a skilled hunter/gatherer at a fast food restaurant, avoid all fried foods, no matter what they are. Those oils are heated and heated and heated again. They become more denatured, unstable, and toxic with each use. There is no life in consuming them. Order grilled, baked, steamed, or boiled food instead. I know you probably know how to do these things, but do you actually do and practice them?

We are made for real food. Meats, dairy, eggs, fish, fruits, vegetables, roots, nuts, seeds - your body knows what to do with these foods. Again, there are always exceptions, and not everything fits into a beautiful box with a bow on top. Allergies and intolerances indicate that you should avoid certain foods. Heed what your body tells you here. You can actually listen to your body regarding all foods. If you eat something, notice how your body feels afterwards. Do you feel good? Energetic? Or, do you feel sick, tired, bloated, achy, etc? Remember, your body is an expression suit. It takes in information (food is information) and it expresses output based on the information you took in. Your intake of food determines your output (expression) to the world. But it also shapes and aligns with your body's inner expressions. The health of your heart, blood vessels, intestines, organs, and all your cells is greatly affected by the nutrients, or lack of nutrients, you put in your mouth.

My only point here is that everything matters. Your thoughts, your actions, your movements, your habits, your food choices - they all contribute to how you interact and express yourself with the world around you. They all answer the question, "Am I safe?" If the answer to that question becomes more "Nos" than "Yesses," we will always be limited to how well we can express and share ourselves with the world.

If everything matters to our body and everything answers the ultimate question constantly being asked, what we eat certainly matters. This means not eating well ultimately stresses our expression suit and drains our ability to live life well. Eating poorly is similar to forgetting to put your mask on first. Poor lifestyle nutritional choices will ultimately limit our effectiveness.

Getting good nutrition and eating healthy food should be simple, but simple does not mean easy, especially in today's world.

You've undoubtedly seen how chaotic and confusing the nutritional scene is now. Nutrition is now treated like religion and politics. People draw lines in the sand about food rules and eating practices. People adopt identities over their food habits. The cows aren't just sacred. They are vilified, abused, and misunderstood. But then, so are the vegetables. To make things worse, you can find a nutritional study that proves or affirms anything you want to see or hear. So what we have now are hosts of studies that cancel one another out. Everyone is right. And while two seemingly opposing things can be true at the same time, it appears that some of our studies have been biased by seeking results that support the desired outcomes rather than attempting to disprove them.

The point is that our plethora of research creates considerable confusion. There is also a ton of information from well-meaning (and perhaps profit-seeking) influencers that further muddies the waters of sound nutrition. Carbs make you fat and cause diabetes. Fat makes you fat and causes diabetes. Plants heal your gut and your body. Plants are trying to kill you; they destroy your gut and wreck your body. The carnivore diet will cure you of all diseases. The carnivore diet will cause inflammation and spark a host of diseases. Low-fat diets cure heart and cholesterol problems. High-fat diets optimize your hormones and protect your brain. Eggs are healthy. Eggs are dangerous. It's an absolute hot mess of confusion out there. But that's what lies do best - they cause chaos and confusion.

So, I'm not going to tell you what you should eat or even suggest that I know what is best for you. I don't. Instead, I'm going to suggest that you eat as if you were in love with your body and you really wanted to take the best care of it. Your body is a gift; it is the vehicle you get to experience the world in, the vehicle you get to express yourself in. Feed your body as if you loved it. And when in doubt, just do the best you can, in faith, with as much understanding of your body's design as you have.

To achieve this, it may be helpful to consider the design of a human being.

When a baby is born, its mother produces milk for it to feed on. There is a need and a supply. The baby needs carbohydrates, proteins, fats, liquids, and nutrients. The mother's body creates all of these things for the child. Just for fun, marinate on that for one second: the mother's body supplies carbohydrates, proteins, and fat for her baby human. These are essential for the child to thrive.

Along with these essential macronutrients and the micronutrients they contain, the mother's love for the child ensures that the child's needs will be met. If it is hungry, her body creates the supply, and she feeds her child. Most mothers would never think of feeding their newborn baby corn syrup, Oreos, Twinkies, potato chips, or any other boxed or bagged food. Most mothers intuitively know that these convenient foods are not what their child needs. Nor are these foods the best sources of nutrients their child should have. They instinctively know their child needs the nutrients their body is supplying.

Yes, eventually the baby grows teeth and becomes able to eat solid foods, but the baby's body still needs the same "rocks" - carbohydrates, proteins, fats, water, and vitamins and minerals. The same is true for the adult. And almost all adults know they shouldn't be feeding themselves with boxed and bagged, hyperpalatable foods. This is why I say we should eat like we actually love ourselves. We should supply our body with the nutrients it is designed to have and the ones it is looking for in their most natural forms, AS BEST WE CAN.

When we really love someone, we give them our best. Our body should be no different. It deserves our best, too. Whether it's our best sources of food, our best decisions about food, or our best intentions - it's worth it to honor our body's design for sustenance. Your body knows what to do with real food. It is designed to consume real food. It is not designed to respond to the lies of modern chemical interpretations or to the imitations of food.

That's it. Eat as if you loved your body. Do the best you can to give it the best you can. Don't get too caught up in the chaos. If Coca-Cola funded the study, it doesn't really matter what the results are. If a drug company is presenting the information, it will probably frame its drug in a positive light. If an influencer is selling a product that seems to be the solution to the study they are highlighting, they may not have your best interests in mind.

Yes, do your own research, but also consider the design of all creation. Everything is supplied for, and everything supplies for the whole. The earth feeds the creatures that live on it. The creatures ultimately return the favor and keep the supply going. Everything "fits" inside the balance of the design, and the design is brilliant. Every time humans try to outsmart our design, we fall short. Our bodies are designed to naturally process real food. We chew, we have enzymes and acids, smooth muscle contractions, and even synergistic relationships with bacteria - all of which come together to break down our food into usable energy and building blocks. Our bodies also nudge us with sensory cues and intuitions on what they need. Though most of us ignore these cues due to all the "noise" and distractions we are surrounded by. We don't have to hunt or gather; we are surrounded by manmade delights that seem to fling themselves at us. But still, we have deep intuitions. Deep down, you likely know that real food is better than Frankenstein foods and fast foods. You can enhance those deep intuitions and bring them to the surface by considering your design and loving your body. What does your body need? What does the Earth provide for you? Do you have a red dye #40 deficiency? Are you depleted in sodium nitrate? Can man-made fats be better for you than fats found in nature?

Your body is intelligent. You are, too. If you want your body to function correctly, feel really good in your body, then love your body, and choose to eat well. As best you can, make real foods the majority of your diet. Within the framework of your food beliefs, if it grows, swims, grazes, blooms, breathes CO_2, breathes O_2 - your body is designed to consume these things. If it is enhanced, chemically preserved, colored, high-heat extruded, packaged, or boxed with cartoon characters and clowns, it may not be the best thing for your body to flourish from. In fact, it may deteriorate your health rather than enhance it.

Food is information. In time, your body expresses its truth or its lies. Just as you don't want to feed your mind with half-truths, lies, and their negativity, you don't want to feed your body with half-foods or fake foods. Yes, some people can live a pretty long time on altered Frankenstein foods, but that doesn't mean they enjoy the quality of vibrant life that is offered with real, wholesome food. It's not just about the mileage we get out of our bodies; it's how we get there. Our bodies are made to thrive. On real food…

TWO THINGS

" There are only two things in life that you worry about: Whether you're healthy or you're sick. If you're healthy, you ain't got nothing to worry about. But if you're sick, you got two things to worry about..."

—COMEDIAN MIKE GOODWIN.

The brain is always asking, "Am I safe?" That's also the same question that our ego is always asking, "Am I safe?" When they both get together and determine that the answer is "No," our thoughts get consumed and hijacked by our own selfishness. When we don't feel safe, when we don't feel whole and well, all we think about is ourselves.

For example, have you ever been injured or in a lot of pain? What did you think about? Likely, your pain. But is that all you thought about? Did you also think about how this pain would affect your life if it didn't end? When you were injured or in pain, did you feel like going out and smiling at everyone you met? Did you feel like fully giving yourself to others who were in need of encouragement, a helping hand, or a favor? Likely, you didn't. It's very hard to think altruistically when we are in pain.

This same self-consumption also happens when we are afraid or overcome by our anxious thoughts. When we fear the boogeyman of time or imagination, we shrink in our expression. We withdraw from the world and become consumed with our fears. They influence how we think, how we interact with others, how we sleep, how we move, etc.

When we are in pain or scared, our world shrinks because our brains and egos fixate on our situation or condition. We become a black hole of self-thought, spiraling deeper and deeper in our imaginative thoughts of doom. To make this worse, remember that our thoughts are one of the chief messengers to the question, "Am I safe?" Our thoughts intensify our pain and fears; we can actually condition our nervous system to be hyper-sensitive to our pains and limitations. But we can also condition our brains to be hyper-ready to dwell on thoughts of fear and doom. This is called obsessing, and it actually alters the neuronal connectivity of the brain, allowing us to obsess over our negative thoughts effortlessly.

The point is, when we hurt, physically or psychologically, our world shrinks into an abyss of self-consumption, and our True Self is lost or hidden from the world.

Conversely, when we feel good in our bodies and in our minds, we feel amazing. When we feel amazing, we don't even think about ourselves at all. Personally, when my body feels amazing, I'm not even aware that I have a body. What I mean is that my body does not distract me from the world when everything in it is functioning correctly. Likewise, when my mind is free from fear, I don't really have any thoughts or "chatter" in my head to distract me from the world; I'm present, tuned in, and alive.

You've likely also experienced this yourself. There have probably been times in your life when you simply felt amazing and joyful - no doubt those were times when you were not consumed with yourself. Those were probably also times when you shared your radiant light with the world and lifted everyone around you.

I am convinced this is how it is supposed to be: we are meant to feel so good that we are oblivious to ourselves but wonderfully evident to everyone around us. And when our brain and our egos know that we are safe, this is how it is - we become selfless. When we become selfless, we become useful, and that's when we are truly alive.

Lose Yourself to Save Yourself

"If you cling to your life, you will lose it, and if you let your life go, you will save it."
—LUKE 17:33, NLT

On the plane, self-preservation is vital as it allows you to help those around you. Putting your oxygen mask on first ensures you are there, able to help others put theirs on as well. That act of self-preservation becomes a selfless act, enabling your life to help preserve the lives around you.

Like in life on the plane, in that emergency, your life has a purpose. It is to be used in the service of others. Immediate emergencies often strip away our selfish orientations. In emergencies, many people often become their True Selves and give their lives to help and save others. Your True Self is selfless. In fact, your True Self is so selfless that if a plane were going down, you may actually try to put someone else's mask on before putting on your own. This is the reason airlines have to tell people to put theirs on first.

The problem with life, though, is that we usually have time to consider ourselves. Our "emergent life" often moves much more slowly than an immediate emergency. In our day-to-day lives, our brains and egos sift through billions of bits of information, trying to determine whether they are safe or not. Along with this sifting, we become imaginative of fears that are not real. Yes, we imagine fears to protect ourselves from them - our brains and egos are clever, in a Spy vs. Spy way. They anticipate and create imagined trouble to perform their jobs of protecting us from the message that we are not safe. Isn't that wild? Anyway, real or imagined fear is treated the same by your brain - it's real.

Your nervous system physically responds to your fearful imagination the same as it would to a real threat. It throws you into fight, flight, or freeze mode - into selfish mode. A lifetime of navigating through real and imagined fear can ultimately dissolve us from our True Self. Instead of being selfless, we become preoccupied with ourselves. Before we know it, we are the black hole of our own alternate universe, creating a reality that consumes everything and everyone for the upside-down gain of feeling safe and secure.

In this alternate reality, we take advantage of people. We ignore people. We hurt people. We don't respect people. We will serve them, but only if it lifts us or serves us in the process.

But on the plane, many of us are stripped of our black-hole, consuming self, and we see someone we love, someone that matters, someone that needs help. On the plane, in a real emergency, many of us would lose ourselves to save another. On the plane, in that emergent moment, we become truly alive.

To be truly alive is to be unencumbered, untethered, and unaware of ourselves. True life is selfless and seeks to give itself away for the sake of another. And in the process of giving itself away, it secures itself.

Jesus once said that there is no greater love than to lay down one's life for one's friend. But there is also no greater feeling than to truly give yourself away. To pour yourself out for another is to be truly alive - to feel amazing, to feel like…Love.

In an immediate emergency, we know this. We do this. We pour our True Self out for the sake of others.

But in the day-to-day, most of us try to make sure we fill and protect our own cup. In the day-to-day, we get hijacked by our fears, our imaginations, our traumas, our injuries, our needs, and our neurology. In our day-to-day lives, many of us lose our lives because we are trying to cling to them.

Clinging to life is the new rage in the "health and fitness" sphere. Longevity and Bio-hacking are all the rage right now because we don't want to die. I would argue that most of the world's problems come from our fear of death. But to say the least, dying is "not safe."

So, thanks to social media and the desire to live forever, we now have a plethora of longevity gurus seeking to outsmart their biology. The wild thing is that many of these gurus are so focused on living forever that they are unable to live in the present. Some of them paint themselves into a rigid corner, or constrain themselves with a myriad of intricate rules and magic levers in an attempt to add years to their lives. I'm not sure they can be successful, though. Something tells me that our days were written and numbered before we ever came into being. That, and there are so many random events in life that are simply outside of our control; each day we have is truly a gift, and nothing that we earn. If anything, our days are gifts we should try to maximize.

Anyway, even if the longevity gurus are successful in adding a day, they are, at the same time, robbing themselves of the very days they want to extend. At best, they are trading immense effort for time; effort that consumes their current time and the one sure thing they actually have: Now. At worst, they are laboring through miserable lives, missing out on the joys of the moments, becoming so consumed with their own bodies and lives that they miss out on sharing their lives with others.

What good is an extra five years if it costs you twenty miserable years to get there? What good is being a lonely centenarian standing in the middle of the memories of the damaged and broken relationships that were traded to get there?

Life is more than time.

It's also more than the vantage point of our personal narrative. The effort to keep the narrative alive above all else can become the act of losing our True Self and our True life, the life we were meant to live. Don't get me wrong, I don't want anyone to ever die, but more than that, I want everyone to truly live, including myself.

Our True life is only found when we are carefree. Free of worries, free of fears, free of pains, free of obsessions, and free of self-awareness. When we are at peace, when we are truly "safe" and oblivious to ourselves, then we are truly alive, and it is only then that our lives truly matter, because when we are truly alive, we become gifts to the world, and that matters. A life that matters is a life that naturally pours itself out to and for others. This is life. This is Love.

In fact, there is no life without Love. But isn't this what Jesus was saying? There is no greater Love than to lay down one's life for one's friends. Love pours itself out; it gives its life away. Without Love, we can do nothing - except be afraid.

Love is the answer to the one question the brain is always asking, "Am I Safe?" It's the antidote to the one fear the ego is always dreading - death. We cannot be safe in the absence of Love. Every child comes into the world in the absence of fear. Love is their default setting - Love is our default setting.

But a child eventually learns to fear. And what soothes the fears of a child? The comforting love of a parent. That love is seen and felt through hugs, words, presence, and devotion. A loving parent often pours themselves out for their child.

When we are not loved, when we don't feel loved, we are not safe. When we are not safe, we don't trust our lives, our world, or our bodies. When we don't feel safe, we are constantly, consciously or subconsciously, looking for ways to feel safe. These ways are often unstable. We look for strength and power, we look for money and wealth, we look for affirmation and being "right," we look for importance, and so on. When we are not safe, our thoughts are inwardly focused, and we become consumers. But we can never consume enough; instead, we drown in our consumption, which is driven by fear.

And that's the rub. Fear keeps us from living. In fact, fear's job is to make sure that we don't live at all. We can exist in time but have no life in us - that's what fear wants.

But that is not our design.

We are designed to truly have life - to be alive, joyful, free, and powerful.

And I can prove it.

Your body is designed to heal and be strong throughout your entire life. Love takes care of its children and their needs. Love designed us to heal through movement. Not only that, but Love also attaches our thoughts and emotions to how well we move. We are clearly designed to move very well; therefore, we are clearly designed to feel very good.

Our very design screams that we are loved.

If we engage with and live in our design at any time, our bodies immediately start working better and eventually work optimally. Now, watch this: living in our design tells our brain we are safe. Our brain is designed to feel and know that it is safe. Safety comes from Love, which crowds out fear.

If our brain is only asking one question, and if the answer to that question determines our expression and our ability to display optimal expression, then we must be made for safety. And if we are made for safety, we have to be made for Love because we can only be safe through Love. And this is how we preserve our lives - we trust in Love.

Trust means we are safe. To be able to trust, we must know that we are loved. If we don't, we can never feel safe; we will always be consumed with our own safety and ourselves. And this is how we end up losing our lives and missing out on experiencing our True Self.

Hear me now, believe me later: We are made to feel amazing. AND, we are loved.

We may not know this or experience this because of fear. Our fear robs us of meaningful, significant lives. Fear causes us to shrink and implode - to be self-consumed. And, to add insult to injury, fear literally makes us weak. But Love urges us to grow, expand, and give ourselves away. It allows us to share our lives with others - to be compassionate. And, because Love provides our safety, it allows us to experience AND express our strength.

This is the key to having a quality of life. Again, it's not about how long we live, it's about how we live. Days and time are not promised; now is all we have. If you want to enjoy a fantastic quality of life and feel amazing, let Love chase your fears away. If that seems too nebulous, start here:

Live in your design: Master breathing, move often, engage in your gait pattern throughout the day.

Get even stronger: Pick things up from the ground, lift things over your head, and carry things for time and distance.

Eat like you actually love yourself.

Consider your design: Ponder how wonderfully made you are, how you're designed to heal, how your brain wants to know you're safe, how freedom of expression comes from feeling safe, and how safety comes from being loved.

If you struggle with this part, I invite you to ask your body what it knows. Test a movement baseline, such as your toe touch or deep squat. Say out loud or in your head, "I am not loved" three times, then test your baseline again. Was it better or worse? Now, say out loud or in your head, "I am loved" three times. Test your baseline now. Was it better or worse? Be honest, your baseline was better when you said, "I am loved." The idea of being loved provides a sense of safety, which makes you move better. OR, your body simply responds to the truth. It shrinks from lies and expands towards truth.

The point is, you are loved.

If you know that, it's like putting your oxygen mask on first. It allows you to fully and freely express yourself by removing the weight and shackles of fear. Knowing you are secure in love truly lightens you. Knowing you are loved preserves your life, reveals your True Self, and allows you to navigate this world with grace and ease. It allows you to reach out and love others, helping to set them free from the lies of their fears.

I know you know that fear is contagious. But so is Love. In fact, Love is the only antidote for fear. Love doesn't just answer the one question your brain, heart, and ego are always asking: "Am I safe?" Love removes the question. And by doing so, you can thrive and live in your highest form, your True Self.

THE ANSWER IS YES

If there is a seemingly perpetual question, there must exist an absolute answer. Your brain is designed to ask, "Am I safe?" Your heart and ego are always asking the same question.

"Am I safe?"

If you are designed to ask that question, and if the answer to that question determines how you give or take from the world, how you will live in your existence, then you must be designed to receive the one answer that has always existed: YES, you are safe.

Love is the YES you have been looking for your whole life. It is the anchor that keeps you safe. You are designed for Love to say "Yes" and resolve that question forever. If you let yourself receive the Yes...

And that's the rub. You have to allow Love to embrace you and remove or resolve your fears. And that is how you put your mask on first: You lose yourself. This is how you slip into the background and place others in the foreground.

You accept that you are loved. No matter what the world says, no matter what your situation says, no matter what your spouse says, no matter what your boss says.

No matter what.

Ultimately, living in your design allows love to hold you and soothe you.

You secure your life, you find your life, when you rest in the Love that holds you. Then, when you are secure in Love, you become oblivious to yourself, and you can give yourself away. This is being truly alive. And it feels terrific.

I apologize if I've lost you. It is just that I've been teaching the wonders of the design of the human body for over fifteen years now, and the more I think I know, the more the wonder keeps revealing itself to me. We are brilliantly and wonderfully designed. We are full of genetic code more complex than we will ever be able to create ourselves. Our bodies never stop growing and evolving; our brains grow and learn throughout our entire lives. We build our brains through our thoughts, movements, and habits. We walk on two feet! We have thumbs! We have emotion, empathy, compassion, and passion. We are full of systems, chemicals, signals, defenses, redundancies, and healing/reparation strategies. We have predicting brains, reflexive bodies, the ability to sprint, to throw, write, and create poems. We can build pyramids, towers, and flying machines. We are filled with and capable of immeasurable wonder. And the secret to experiencing all that wonder is hidden in our very bodies.

Like begets like, so Wonder begets wonder.

And when you get a glimpse of how the wonder works, of how we can even use that wonder to our advantage, it changes everything. It can even set you free.

The point is, we are never stuck. If we are stuck, it is only because we have chosen the lies of fear. But fear creates suffering, and we are not meant for the sufferings of fear; we are meant for the joys of Love.

I titled this book Self-Preservation, but that is somewhat misleading. It's not about preserving our identities or beliefs about ourselves, as much as it is about removing them and living as our True selves, experiencing our true potential.

In a sense, my version of self-preservation is precisely the opposite of conventional self-preservation. It's self-realization, finding the abundance of life rather than the scarcity of life.

We do this by sending the constant message of "Yes, I am safe" to our brain, our heart, and our ego. This happens through renewing our minds and thoughts, moving and breathing through our foundational, predetermined movement patterns, and using our bodies to engage in challenging practices. Experiencing our design opens the doors of wonder. This wonder can ultimately lead us to discovering the most enormous YES to safety: Love.

To review, Love washes away fear. It removes or satisfies the question of "Am I safe?" This allows us to explode into the world rather than implode into ourselves.

But don't believe me. Test this out for yourself.

Experience your design; breathe and move the way you were born to, and experience how much better you move and feel. Practice and perfect your strength by challenging it by moving, lifting, and carrying heavy things. Experience your thoughts by harnessing them on positive, useful things and protecting them from negative, harmful things.

And finally, set out to experience Love. Practice receiving it, allowing it, and accepting it. Test how your body (your movements) and your mind (your thoughts) respond to it. Test how thoughts of fear make you move and feel, and contrast that with how thoughts of being loved make you move and feel. Experiment and experience it. Then ponder why and how this all works and happens the way it does. Let your experience guide you towards the truth:

You are safe.

Because you are loved.

LEARN MORE ABOUT ORIGINAL STRENGTH

Original Strength Systems (OS) is the leader in nervous system restoration and development of reflexive strength or functional movement. Our mission is to bring the hope and strength of movement to every body in the world. We provide accredited continuing education courses and books for health, fitness, and education professionals, empowering them to deliver better outcomes to their patients, clients, athletes, and students.

Based on the human developmental sequence, a series of movements that all humans naturally go through as they grow, and the human body's design, OS's Pressing RESET method teaches movements that help RESET an individual's neuromuscular system, allowing them to enjoy improved physical movement and physiological function.

If you want to learn more about Pressing RESET and reclaiming your original strength, https://originalstrength.net is your gateway.

There, you'll discover a wealth of resources, from comprehensive books to hundreds of free video tutorials (OS Movemen Snaxs), Pressing RESET: Original Strength Forever, and a complete directory of our courses and OS Certified Professionals in your vicinity. We're here to support you every step of the way.

When you're ready to enhance your movement system, we encourage you to connect with an OS Certified Professional. They can conduct an Original Strength Screen and Assessment (OSSA), a quick and straightforward method to identify areas for improvement. With the OSSA, the professional can guide you to the most effective starting point for your journey to restore your Original Strength through the Pressing RESET technique.

Remember, the OS team is always here for you. If you have any questions or need further guidance, please don't hesitate to reach out.

We're committed to your journey towards better movement and health. Please keep us updated on your progress. We want to know how you are doing. Progress@OriginalStrength.net

"...I am fearfully and wonderfully made..."
—PSALM 139:14

www.ingramcontent.com/pod-product-compliance
Lightning Source LLC
Chambersburg PA
CBHW051326120626
46547CB00015B/2419